HEPATITIS B VIRUS
RESEARCH FOCUS

HEPATITIS B VIRUS RESEARCH FOCUS

XIAODONG ZHANG, WEIYING ZHANG AND LIHONG YE

Nova Biomedical Books
New York

Library of Congress Cataloging-in-Publication Data

Zhang, Xiaodong, 1970-
  Hepatitis B virus research focus / Xiaodong Zhang, Weiying Zhang, Lihong Ye (authors).
    p. ; cm.
  Includes bibliographical references.
  ISBN 978-1-60456-299-6 (softcover)
  1. Hepatitis B virus. I. Zhang, Weiying, 1968- II. Ye, Lihong. III. Title.
  [DNLM: 1. Hepatitis B--drug therapy. 2. Hepatitis B--prevention & control. 3. Hepatitis B virus. WC 536 Z625h 2008]
  QR201.H46Z43   2008
  616.3'623--dc22   2008019727

Published by Nova Science Publishers, Inc. ✤ *New York*

Contents

Preface

Hepatitis B virus (HBV), discovered in 1966, infects more than 350 million people in the world. The infection of HBV is a leading cause of chronic carriage of the virus and progressive liver diseases, such as hepatitis, liver cirrhosis and hepatocellular carcinoma (HCC). HBV consists of a circular, partially double-stranded DNA molecule of 3.2 kb in length, which contains four overlapping reading frames that code for surface proteins (HBsAg), core proteins (HBcAg/HBeAg), the viral polymerase, and the transcriptional transactivator X protein. Chronic hepatitis appears to be due to a suboptimal cellular immune response that destroys some of the infected hepatocytes and does not purge the virus from the remaining infected hepatocytes, thereby permitting the persisting virus to trigger a chronic indolent necroinflammatory liver disease that sets the stage for development of HCC. However, the mechanisms responsible for malignant transformation in chronic HBV infection are not well defined, and both viral and host factors have been implicated in the process. All cases of HCC occur after many years of chronic hepatitis which could, theoretically, provide the mitogenic and mutagenic environment to precipitate random genetic and chromosomal damage, and lead to the development of HCC. Hepatitis B virus X protein (HBx), an important transforming inducer, plays a crucial role in HCC development. HBx has the capability to influence a variety of signal transduction pathways within the cells. Monitoring of the HBV genotypes and antibody to Hepatitis B x antigen (anti-HBx) are significant for predicting early diagnosis of liver cirrhosis and HCC. HBV and Hepatitis C virus or HIV coinfections can accelerate the course of chronic liver disease and facilitate progression to cirrhosis and HCC. As for therapy of liver diseases, five drugs are now FDA-approved for the treatment of HBV, including interferon (IFN), lamivudine, adefovir, entecavir, and peginterferon alfa-2a. Moreover, the prevention for HBV infection is very important. It is likely that the most important outcome of the research on HBV has been the invention, development, and application of the vaccine against HBV. However, at present most investigators focus on basic research rather than practical applications. The HBV research should be focused on animal models and clinical practice. The technology update in HBV research and the multisubject combination may be attached importance to next a few decades. Some molecular approaches, such as antisense, oligonucleotides, ribozymes, RNA interference targeting HBV mRNA, are available in antiviral therapies.

Chapter I

Molecular Epidemiology

Hepatitis B virus (HBV), discovered in 1966, infects more than 350 million people in the world. The infection of HBV is a leading cause of chronic hepatitis B (CHB), liver cirrhosis (LC), and hepatocellular carcinoma (HCC), accounting for one million deaths annually. Chronic HBV patients can fluctuate between periods of active liver inflammation and periods of inactive disease.

Disease progression can be influenced by various factors [1]. Genetic factors not only influence host response to HBV infection, but also affect the response to CHB vaccine. Substantial genetic epidemiology studies indicate that HBV spreads in the families. The familial occurrence of HBV infection has been well established in some ethnic groups. Ohbayashi *et al* 2] have reported 3 Japanese families in which 36 of the 54 members are HBsAg positive. Of these, some are healthy carriers while others have liver cirrhosis and hepatocellular carcinoma. Similar observations have been reported in American [3], European [4] and Asian [5, 6] continents. This observed familial clustering may stem from inherited defects in specific genes, from shared environmental exposures among family members or from interaction between specific genetic and environmental factors. These studies have provided important insights into the fact that different ethnics in the same region have different HBV epidemiological characteristics and the same races in the different region share the same prevalence of HBV markers, indicating that genetic factors may play a role in maintaining the frequency of HBV infection and persistence. Moreover, molecular epidemiology study has identified several genetically determined differences among races.

Analysis of genetic susceptibility to HBV infection aims to link these DNA variations (the genotype) with a particular HBV infection (the phenotype). HBV infection and clearance are complex traits [7], meaning that the genetic contribution to them is not inherited in a exert effects on the outcome [8]. Many possible approaches to mapping the genes underlying complex traits fall broadly into two categories: candidate gene- based association studies and genome-wide linkage studies [9].

Hepatitis B virus is present in the blood, saliva, semen, vaginal secretions, menstrual blood, and to a lesser extent, perspiration, breast milk, tears, and urine of infected individuals. A highly resilient virus, HBV is resistant to breakdown, can survive outside the body, and is easily transmitted through contact with infected body fluids. Transmission occurs *via* perinatal, sexual, and parenteral routes, particularly intravenous drug abuse and although blood products still carry a risk, this is now extremely low in western countries. In areas of high endemicity, the most common route of transmission is perinatal or the infection is acquired during the preschool years. In areas of intermediate endemicity, transmission is either perinatal or horizontal [10,11]. The route of transmission has important clinical implications, because there is a very high probability of developing CHB if the infection is acquired perinatally or in the preschool years [12]. The use of unsafe injections poses a particular public health problem in the developing countries [13]. Contaminated needles cause 8–16 million HBV infections each year, compared with 2.3–4.7 million hepatitis C virus infections, and 80,000–160,000 human immunodeficiency virus infections [14]. In areas of low endemicity, most HBV infections are acquired by horizontal transmission in early adult life, i.e. through intravenous drug use or unprotected sexual activities [11]. Blood transfusions were once a common route of transmission, but improved diagnostic tests and progressively broader screening for HBV infection in recent years, such as occurred in Latin American countries from 1994 to 1997, has dramatically reduced the risk of acquiring HBV infection through transfusion [15]. Other sources of infection include contaminated surgical instruments and donor organs. Health care workers, dentists, and others who have frequent contact with infected blood or blood products are at highest risk.

Only a minority of infected adult cases is able to develop chronic hepatitis but in children under 1 year, 90% develop chronic hepatitis [16]. About one forth of them will develop chronic hepatitis and cirrhosis and could develop hepatocellular carcinoma eventually. The probability of becoming a chronic carrier is inversely related to age at the time of infection [17]. Although only 5–10% of adults infected with HBV will become chronic carriers, neonatal infection almost always leads to a chronic carrier state (90%) whereas 30–60% of children infected during the first five years of life will become chronic HBV carriers [18]. The precise mechanism of this has not yet been defined but it has been attributed to the immaturity of the immune system of newborns and young children and their inability to mount an effective CTL response against HBV infection [19,20]. Acute and chronic HBV infections are usually asymptomatic during childhood. Up to 25% of infants and older children who acquire chronic HBV infection will eventually develop HBV-related hepatocellular carcinoma or cirrhosis.

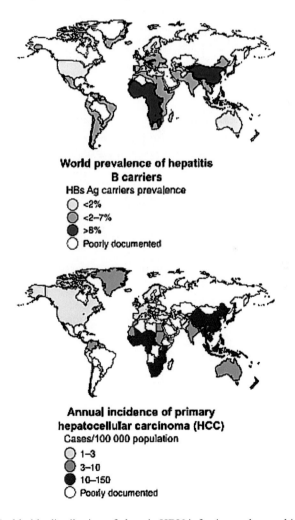

World prevalence of hepatitis B carriers
HBs Ag carriers prevalence
○ <2%
◔ <2–7%
● >8%
○ Poorly documented

Annual incidence of primary hepatocellular carcinoma (HCC)
Cases/100 000 population
○ 1–3
◔ 3–10
● 10–150
○ Poorly documented

Figure 1.1. Worldwide distribution of chronic HBV infection and annual incidence of primary hepatocellular carcinoma (HCC).

The distribution of HBV infection varies greatly throughout the world. The prevalence of HBV infection varies markedly in different geographic areas of the world, as well as in different population subgroups (figure 1) [21].

Overall, approximately 45% of the global population lives in areas of high chronic HBV prevalence [22]. The prevalence is high in some areas, such as Southeast Asia, China, and Africa. In sub-Saharan Africa, the Pacific, and particularly Asia, HBV infection is highly endemic, with the majority of individuals becoming infected during childhood. Outside of the endemic areas, regions with high rates of chronic HBV infection include the southern parts of Eastern and Central Europe, the Amazon basin, the Middle East, and the Indian subcontinent. Areas with low levels of endemicity include North America, Western Europe, and Australia. In western and northern European countries and North America, HBV infection is relatively rare and acquired primarily in adulthood [23]. Regions with a high prevalence of HBV infection also have high rates of HCC (figure 1). HBV causes 60–80% of the world's primary liver cancer, one of the three major causes of death in Asia, the Pacific Rim and Africa (Table 1) [24, 25]. In both high- and low-incidence areas, HCC predominates in males, with male-to-female ratios of 3–4 to 1.

References

[1]   McMahon BJ. (2005). Epidemiology and natural history of hepatitis B. *Semin. Liver Dis*, 25 (Suppl 1):3-8.

[2]   Obayashi A, Okochi K, Mayumi M. (1972).Familial clustering of asymptomatic carriers of Australia antigen and patients with chronic liver disease or primary liver cancer. *Gastroenterology*, 62: 618-625.

[3]   Motta-Castro AR, Martins RM, Yoshida CF, Teles SA, Paniago AM, Lima KM, Gomes SA.(2005).Hepatitis B virus infection in isolated Afro-Brazilian communities. *J. Med. Virol*, 77: 188-193.

[4]   Bosch J, Brugera M, Rodes J. (1973). Familial spread of type-B hepatitis. *Lancet*, 2: 457.

[5]   Beasley RP, Hwang LY, Stevens CE, Lin CC, Hsieh FJ, Wang KY, Sun TS, Szmuness W.(1983). Efficacy of hepatitis B immune globulin for prevention of perinatal transmission of the hepatitis B virus carrier state: fi nal report of a randomized double-blind, placebo-controlled trial. *Hepatology* , 3: 135-141.

[6]   Lin JB, Lin DB, Chen SC, Chen PS, Chen WK.(2006). Seroepidemiology
       of hepatitis A, B, C, and E viruses infection among preschool children in
       Taiwan. *J. Med. Virol*, 78: 18-23.

[7]   Thursz M. (2004).Pros and cons of genetic association studies in hepatitis
       B. *Hepatology*, 40: 284-286.

[8]   Newton-Cheh C, Hirschhorn JN. (2005) Genetic association studies of
       complex traits: design and analysis issues. *Mutat. Res*, 573: 54-69.

[9]   Hirschhorn JN, Daly MJ. (2005).Genome-wide association studies for
       common diseases and complex traits. *Nat. Rev. Genet*, 6:95-108.

[10]   Lok AS. (2002).Chronic hepatitis B. *N. Engl. J. Med*, 346(22):1682–1683.

[11]   Gust ID.(1996).Epidemiology of hepatitis B infection in the Western
       Pacific and South East Asia. *Gut*, 38(Suppl 2): S18–23.

[12]   Chen CJ, Wang LY, Yu MW.(2000).Epidemiology of hepatitis B virus
       infection in the Asia-Pacific region. *J. Gastroenterol. Hepatol*;
       15(Suppl.): E3–6.

[13]   Simonsen L, Kane A, Lloyd J et al.(1999).Unsafe injections in the
       developing world and transmission of blood borne pathogens: a review.
       Bull. World Health Organ, 77(10): 789–800.

[14]   Kane A, Lloyd J, Zaffran M et al. (1999). Transmission of hepatitis B,
       hepatitis C and human immunodeficiency viruses through unsafe
       injections in the developing world: model-based regional estimates. *Bull
       World Health Organ*, 77(10):801–807.

[15]   Schmunis GA, Zicker F, Cruz JR, Cuchi P.(2001).Safety of blood supply
       for infectious diseases in Latin American countries, 1994–1997. *Am. J.
       Trop. Med. Hyg* , 65(6):924–930.

[16]   Walsh K, Alexander GJ. (2001). Update on chronic viral hepatitis.
       Postgrad Med. J , 77 (910), 498-505.

[17]   Hyams KC.(1995).Risks of chronicity following acute hepatitis B virus
       infection; a review. *Clin. Infect. Dis*, 20:992-1000.

[18]   McMahon BJ, Alward WLM, Hall DB, Heyward WL, Bender TR, Francis
       DP, Maynard JE.(1985). Acute hepatitis B virus infection: relation of age
       to the clinical expression of disease and subsequent development of the
       carrier state. *J. Infect. Dis*, 151:599-603.

[19]   Hsu HY, Chang MH, Ni YH, Lee PI.(1999).Cytokine release of peripheral
       blood mononuclear cells in children with chronic hepatitis B virus
       infection. *JPGN*, 29:540-545.

[20] Hsu HY, Chang MH, Hsieh KH, Lee CY, Lin HH, Hwang LH, Chen PJ, Chen DS.(1992).Cellular Immune response to HBcAg in mother-toinfant transmission of hepatitis B virus. *Hepatology*,14: 770-776.

[21] Yu MC, Yuan JM, Govindarajan S, Ross RK.(2000).Epidemiology of hepatocellular carcinoma. *Can. J. Gastroenterol*, 14(8):703–709.

[22] Mahoney FJ.(1999) Update on diagnosis, management, and prevention of hepatitis B virus infection. *Clin. Microbiol. Rev*,12(2): 351–366.

[23] Lok AS, Heathcote EJ, Hoofnagle JH. (2001). Management of hepatitis B: 2000 – summary of a workshop. *Gastroenterology*,120(7): 1828–1853.

[24] McGlynn KA, Tsao L, Hsing AW, et al. (2001).International trends and patterns of primary liver cancer. *Int. J. Cancer*, 94(2): 290–296.

[25] Lemon SM, Layden TJ, Seeff L, et al.(2000).The 20th United States-Japan Joint Hepatitis Panel Meeting. *Hepatology*, 31(3): 800–806.

Chapter II

Virologic Characteristics

1. Virologic Basic

HBV is the prototype member of the hepadnaviridae family and consists of a circular partially double-stranded DNA molecule of 3.2 kb in length which contains four overlapping reading frames that code for surface proteins (HBsAg), core proteins (HBcAg/HBeAg), the viral polymerase, and the transcriptional transactivator X protein. The S and C genes have upstream regions termed preS and preC (figure 1).

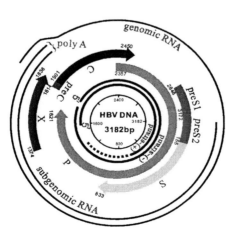

Figure 2.1. Structure of HBV genome. The genome of HBV is a double-stranded circular DNA (3.2 kb), which contains four ORF coding for polymerase (P), surface antigens (PreS1, PreS2, and S), precore (preC), core (C), and X.

The S-gene (NT 2848 to NT 833; type ayw3) codes a 226 amino acid (aa) of protein, named major antigen. The preS2 gene codes a 55 aa protein, which together with the previous major antigen form the medium antigen. The preS1 gene codes a 108 aa protein which together with the previous medium antigen form the large antigen. The C-gene (NT 1814 to NT 2450) codes the core protein (HBcAg) which is a part of the viral nucleocapsid or the HBe antigen which is secerned into the blood, respectively. The X (NT 1374 to NT 1836) open reading frame encodes the viral X protein which modulates host-cell signal transduction and can directly and indirectly affect host and viral gene expression [1]. The P-gene (NT 2307 to NT 1621) codes the viral polymerase (figure 1).

2. Open Reading Frames (ORFs) of HBV

2.1. The S-Gene

The S-gene contains of 3 regions and encodes for 3 different glycoproteins which only differ in the length of their N-terminus. The gene products are designated the s (small)-HBsAg (or major-HBsAg) (226 aa) - encoded only from the S-region -, the m (medium)-HBsAg (281 aa) - encoded from the pre-S2-region and the S-region - and the l (large)-HBsAg (400 or 389 aa depending on subtype) -encoded from the pre-S1-region, the pre-S2-region and the S-region [2].

2.2. The C-Gene

The C-gene contains of two regions. The core region (183 aa) encodes for the viral nucleocapsid (HBc-antigen) and the precore-region (29 aa) together with the core-region for the HBe-antigen which is secreted into the blood. After being processed at its N-terminus and its C-terminus the ripe HBe protein generally contains of the aa 20-29 of the precore-sequence and of the aa 1-149 of the core-sequence [3-6]. An other HBeAg which in addition to the normal HBe-sequence contained the aa 1-19 of the precore-region could be detected [6]. Because the HBsAg preS1 region correlates with the assembly and infectivity of HBV [7], possesses the binding site with hepatocyte membrane [8], has abundant T- and B-cell epitopes [9] and may overcome the noneresponse against the common vaccines containing only S region [10], the incorporation of preS1 region into the epitope-based vaccines has been accepted widely [11,12]. While the incorporate site and size of preS1 sequence are controversial. Some results showed that the immunogenic domains mainly existed in preS1 (21–59) in N-terminus and preS1 (95–109) in C-terminus, and more importantly, a major immunogenic domain preS1 (34–59), which has much stronger immunogenicity, was identified. It was also supported by the predictions of secondary structure and immunological property in the preS1 (21–119) region. The results here would be helpful for the design of new vaccines against HBV.

2.3. The P-Gene

The P-ORF encodes for a multifunctional enzyme (831 aa; 93 kDa) which is called the polymerase (Pol). The polymerase is responsible for the reverse transcription of the pregenomic RNA to the double stranded DNA. Four different domains within the P-gene product could be distinguished (figure 2) [13-15]. The terminal protein is considered to be the part of the polymerase where the synthesis of the minus strand-DNA is initiated. First the terminal protein binds covalently a T. This T will be the 5′terminus of the minus-strand which has been mapped to NT1827 [16]. Interestingly in experiments the human polymerase was able to accept all of the four nucleotides as the first base of the minus-strand. If the terminal protein covalently binds a G then the 5′terminus of the minus-strand may result to be G 1826. This is consistent with the observation that the 5′terminus of the minus-strand was mapped to T 1827 and to G 1826 [17]. However, the strength of the protein-nucleotide-interaction was found to be decreasing from T to G to A to C [212]. This order corresponds to the nucleotid sequence (A, NT1827; C, NT 1826; U, NT 1825) within the DR1. Once synthesized the whole minus-strand-DNA remains protein-bound with its 5′ terminus [18].

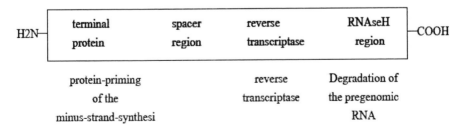

Figure 2.2. Structure and functions of the polymerase.

In the duck-HBV the first nucleotide of the minus-strand (dGMP) is bound to the OH-group of Tyr-96, a part of the terminal protein, by a phosphodiester [19]. Depending on the template also other nucleotides can be accepted by Tyr-96 [20]. Tyr-96 was described to be indispensible for the enzyme function. Furthermore a functional reverse transcriptase region also seems to be required for the priming activity of the duck polymerase [19].

2.4. The X-Gene

Hepatitis B virus X gene (HBx) can be divided into 6 domains (A-F). The C-terminus of the protein (domains C-E) seems to be the transactivating portion [21] while the N terminus of HBx (domain A) can repress the HBx transactivation. Thereby, the N-terminus is believed to avoid an excessive HBx transactivation and to play a role in a self-regulatory mechanism of X gene expression [22]. The various domains of HBx show a very different degree of conservation among mammalian hepadnaviruses (see Table 1). Interestingly the highly conserved domains A, C and E contain the 4 conserved cysteines 7, 61, 69 and 137 [21]. HBx is considered to be unable to bind directly to DNA [23, 24]. However an intrinsic serine/threonine protein kinase activity could be detected [25]. This might imply that the transactivating activity of HBx depends on eukaryotic transcription factors. HBx was found to act in the cytosol and in the nucleus. Various gene regulating pathways of HBx were described.

3. Genotypes

3.1. HBV Genotypes

DNA sequencing of many isolates of HBV has confirmed the existence of 8 viral genotypes, (A-H) [26-29] each with a characteristic geographic distribution (as show in Table 2) [30]: Genotypes of A–D [29] differ by more than 8% at the nucleotide level. Later, genotypes F [31] and E [27] were reported. HBV genotypes G [32, 34] and H were described [33]. Some methods have been developed and used for HBV genotyping including direct sequencing, restriction fragment length polymorphism, line probe assay, enzyme-linked immunoassay and nested PCR. Compared to genotype A, the genotypes B, C, D, E, F, and G have a 6 nucleotide-deletion at the C-terminus of the core gene, in genotype G 36 nucleotides are inserted in the N-terminus of the core-gene [32], while genotype D has a 33 nucleotide-deletion at the N-terminus of the pre-S1-region, and genotypes E and G have a 3 nucleotide-deletion at the N-terminus of the pre-S1-region.

Several studies have evaluated the molecular epidemiology and the relevance of HBV genotypes on clinical outcome. Thus, HBV genotype A appears to be the predominant genotype among patients with HBV infection in North America, Northwest Europe and the sub-saharan Africa, while HBV genotype B and C are frequently found in China and Japan, and HBV genotype D is prevalent in South Europe, Middle East and India [34,35]. Among the eight genotypes, genotype-C is closely related to HCC in Asia. HBV genotype F has been reported in Central and South America [36-38]. The recently discovered type G was found in France and in the USA [32].

Most of these studies have evaluated patients with chronic HBV infection and there are only a few studies that have analyzed the HBV genotype distribution in patients with acute hepatitis B. One study in Switzerland found that genotype A was more common among patients with chronic hepatitis B, whereas genotype D was more prevalent among patients with resolving acute hepatitis B [39].

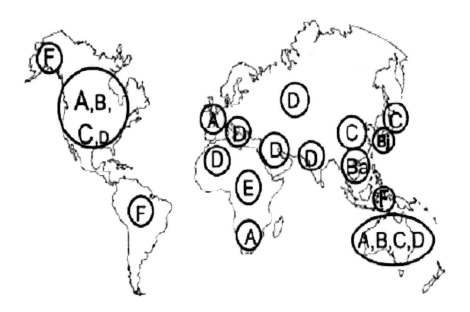

Figure 2.3. Geographic distribution of hepatitis B virus genotypes.

And although there is no clear relationship between HBV genotype and clinical course, they seem to affect disease profile, with a higher chance of viral clearance and sustained remission for patients infected with genotype A than for those infected with genotype D. Figure 3 illustrates the geographic distribution of HBV genotypes, but existing information is incomplete, as data in many parts of the world are not available or are based on very small numbers of patients studied.

3.2. HBV Subgenotypes

Recent works have shown that HBV genotypes can be further segregated into subgenotypes (Table 3) [40-45]. Sugauchi et al. [40] reported that two subgenotypes of genotype B can be differentiated: a Japanese subgenotype Bj and an Asian subgenotype called Ba. Kramvis et al. [42] also found African isolates of genotype A, which showed several interesting features, like a deletion of amino acids 1–11 in preS1 as in genotype D. Sequencing of HBV isolates from Australian Aborigines showed that some of the patients harbored an HBV isolate of genotype C that showed several features of a separate subgenotype called genotype Caustralia [41]. The South American genotype F segregates into two clades: F1 and F2 [44]. Recently, Norder et al. [45] collected sequences of 234 complete genomes and 631 hepatitis B surface genes to assess the worldwide diversity of HBV. Apart from the two subgenotypes described each for A and F, also B, C, and D were divided into four subgenotypes each in the analysis of complete genomes, supported by significant bootstrap values (Table 2). The subgenotypes of B and C differed in their geographical distribution with B1 (Bj) dominating in Japan, B2 (Ba) in China and Vietnam, B3 confined to Indonesia, and B4 confined to Vietnam. Subgenotype C1 (Cs) was common in Japan, Korea, and China; C2 (Ce) in China, South-East Asia, and Bangladesh; C3 in the Oceania; and C4 is encountered in Aborigines from Australia. This pattern of defined geographical distribution was less evident for D1–D4, where the subgenotypes were widely spread in Europe, Africa, and Asia.

3.3. HBV Genotypes, HBeAg Seroconversion and Outcome of Chronic HBV Infection

Most of the information on the clinical significance of HBV genotypes has been based on studies of patients with chronic HBV infection in Asia. Because of the preponderance of genotypes B and C in Asian countries, the studies are restricted to comparisons of patients with these two genotypes. Nevertheless, such comparisons provide very important information on the relation between HBV genotype B and C and the rate of progression of liver disease, since the age at the onset of infection is presumed to be the same (perinatal period) in the vast majority of patients. These studies clearly showed that compared to genotype C, HBV genotype B is associated with spontaneous HBeAg seroconversion at a younger age, less active liver disease, and a slower rate of progression to cirrhosis.[46-51] Some studies also found that genotype B patients are less likely to have hepatitis flares and more likely to remain in remission after HBeAg seroconversion. [51] Most studies, including those outside of Japan, reported that hepatocellular carcinoma (HCC) development is less frequent and occurs at an older age in patients with genotype B. [49,50,52] These data indicate that a shorter duration of high levels of HBV replication and less active necroinflammation may contribute to a more favorable outcome among patients with genotype B.

There is a paucity of data on the clinical course of patients with genotypes other than B and C. One study from Spain reported that HBeAg seroconversion rates were similar in patients with genotypes A and D, but sustained biochemical and virological remission was more common in patients with genotype A who had HBeAg seroconversion. [53] Patients with genotype A also had a higher rate of HBsAg clearance. However, the need for liver transplantation and the deaths related to liver disease were comparable between patients with genotypes A and D. In this study, patients with genotype F were more likely to die from liver disease than those with genotypes A or D, but only 19 patients with genotype F were included.

To date there has been no published study comparing the rate of HBeAg seroconversion, activity of liver disease, and rate of progression to cirrhosis and HCC among patients with all known HBV genotypes. The lack of such studies is related to the preponderance of 1 or 2 HBV genotypes in most geographical regions. The finding of HBV genotypes A to G in the United States permits studies that compare the clinical course of HBV infection among patients with a wider spectrum of HBV genotypes. In one cross-sectional study of 694 patients in the United States, genotypes B and D were associated with a lower prevalence of HBeAg than genotype A, while genotype B was associated with a lower rate of hepatic decompensation compared to genotype A, C, or D. [34] However, other factors such as differences in ethnic/racial background, age at onset and duration of infection, and exposures to alcohol/ environmental toxins rather than HBV genotypes may have contributed to the differences in clinical manifestations.

3.4. HBV Genotypes and Outcome of Acute HBV Infection

There is very little information on the correlation between HBV genotypes and the outcome of acute HBV infection. One study of 65 patients in Switzerland found that 80% of patients with acute hepatitis B had genotype D, while 80% patients with chronic hepatitis B had genotype A. [39] Another study found that 12% of 531 Japanese patients with chronic HBV infection had genotype B in contrast to 39% of 61 patients with acute hepatitis B. [54] These data suggest that different HBV genotypes may be associated with different rates of progression from acute to chronic HBV infection. Alternatively, the data may indicate a temporal change in predominant HBV genotype due to immigration or a shift in mode of transmission.

In summary, there is increasing evidence that HBV genotype correlates with clinical outcomes of chronic HBV infection and response to treatment. The evidence for a clinical difference is stronger between genotypes B and C, and in response to IFN but not nucleoside or nucleotide treatment. The exact reason(s) why HBV genotype may be related to clinical outcomes is not clear. It is possible that different genotypes may be associated with differences in replication fitness and expression of immune epitopes. There is also a clear association between HBV genotypes and precore and core promoter mutations. While the story of HBV genotypes continues to unfold at a rapid pace, genotyping should remain a research tool until the time when knowledge of the HBV genotype can be used to predict the risk of adverse outcomes (fulminant hepatitis, cirrhosis, or HCC) or to guide treatment decisions (choice or duration of therapy).

Clinical manifestations of persistent HBV infection with distinct genotypes. Prospective, case-controlled and cross-sectional studies predominantly but not entirely indicate that the severity and outcome of chronic hepatitis B are more serious in patients infected with genotype C compared with B. [50,55-57] Liver cirrhosis and HCC are more frequent in carriers of genotype C than B. [55,58-60] Very recently, chronic liver disease was detected more frequently in Japanese individuals infected with genotype C than D [221/350(63%) compared with 6/38 (16%), P < 0.001].[61].

To a lesser extent, clinical differences between genotype A and D infections have been reported from Europe, where these genotypes are frequent. HBV infection is contracted in adulthood in these countries, principally through sexual contacts and illicit drug use, and HBV infection is more likely to persist in persons infected with genotype A rather than D or the other genotypes. [39] These findings stand at variance with those of Sanchez-Tapias et al. [53] who found sustained biochemical remission and clearance of HBV DNA to be more frequent in infection with genotype A than genotype D (log-rank, 14.2, P = 0.002) or genotype F (log-rank, 4.2, P = 0.03); the rate of HBsAg clearance was also found to be higher in genotype A compared with D infection (log-rank, 4.06, P = 0.03). Likewise in a comparison between 60 and 63 patients in India infected with HBV genotype A or D, respectively, genotype D was significantly associated with severe liver disease (61% compared with 30%, P < 0.05) and tended to be more frequent in those with HCC below 40 years of age (63% compared with 44%, P = 0.06). [62]

3.5. Influence of HBV Genotype on the Response to Antiviral Therapy

Until lamivudine was developed for clinical use, interferon had remained the sole practical antiviral for chronic hepatitis B, ever since initial clinical trials by Hoofnagle and colleagues [63,64] in the mid-1980s. The response to interferon, judged by the loss of HBeAg from serum, is achieved in at most 20% of treated patients. [65] Moreover, Asian patients who have acquired the HBV carrier state at birth or in early infancy respond to interferon more poorly than Caucasian patients who contracted it in adulthood. To make matters even worse, patients with chronic hepatitis B positive for anti-HBe antibodies are much less responsive to interferon than those with serum HBeAg. Limited experience indicates that HBV genotypes make a difference in the response to interferon in patients with chronic hepatitis B.

Zhang et al. [66] found the response to interferon was higher in patients infected with genotype A compared with D or E (70% versus 40%, P = 0.001). Likewise, Kao et al. [67] reported the response to interferon to be higher in patients infected with genotype B rather than C [13/32 (41%) versus 4/26 (15%), P = 0.045]. More recently, Wai et al. [68] compared the response between patients randomized to interferon or placebo. They found the response was better in patients with genotype B than C infection who were allocated to interferon treatment [12/31 (39%) versus 7/42 (17%), P = 0.034]; the response rate did not differ in those who received placebo.

Lamivudine [(–)-b-L-20, 30-dideoxy-30-thiacytidine] is a nucleoside analogue with a potent antiviral activity. Since its approval in 1998, lamivudine has gained wide popularity for the treatment of chronic hepatitis B due to high a efficacy with minimal untoward effects. [69-73] Chien et al.[74] reported that the sustained response to lamivudine was much higher in patients infected with genotype B compared with genotype C [38/62 (61%) versus 5/20 (20%), P = 0.009].

HBV genotypes influence the severity of liver disease and response to interferon and lamivudine. They are also expected to influence the response to adefovir dipivoxil, which has recently been approved for treatment of chronic hepatitis B, [75] as well as the emergence of resistant mutants; [76] although as yet no differences have been observed in the response to adefovir dipivoxil in relation to HBV genotypes.[77] Should poor responses to a given antiviral be predicted in patients infected with HBV of certain genotypes, they can be directed to the other therapeutic options to spare the cost and burden of treatment. Accumulating evidence indicates a better sustained response to conventional interferon in patients with genotype B than those with C, and in patients with genotype A than those with D. In contrast, conflicting results exist regarding the response to pegylated interferon. On the other hand, the therapeutic responses to nucleoside/nucleotide analogues are comparable among patients with different HBV genotypes. The impact of HBV subgenotypes, mixed genotype infections, and recombinants of different genotypes on the response to antiviral treatments awaits further examinations.

4. Serologic Features

The first stage is characterized by the presence of HBsAg, HBeAg, and IgM class of anti-HBc antibodies, and may last for decades. In the intermediate stage, patients lose HBeAg, develop anti-HBe antibodies, and often enter into clinical remission. Finally, loss of HBsAg and rise of the anti-HBs antibody indicate recovery from infection. With the cloning of the HBV genome, it became apparent that the viremia titer (number of infectious virus particles) is the highest during the HBeAg phase of infection, declines by several logs during the anti-HBe phase, and disappears at the anti-HBs phase.

4.1. Three Viral Antigens

Molecular cloning and sequencing of the HBV genome led to the redefinition of the three HBV antigens as viral gene products endowed with specific functions in viral life cycle. The HBsAg is the envelope protein of the virus, and actually comprises three co-terminal proteins (large, middle, and small) due to the presence of multiple transcripts and alternative translation initiation sites in the gene. They contain preS1/preS2/S domains, preS2/S domains, and S domain, respectively. The small envelope protein, composed of S domain alone, is the most abundantly expressed. The envelope proteins interact with the nucleocapsid to initiate its envelopment, and the resultant virus particle (virion) is released into the bloodstream. Thus, HBcAg is not detectable in patient blood unless the envelope is removed. In addition to their incorporation into virus particles, the envelope proteins can be secreted alone as non-infectious subviral particles, which constitute the bulk of HBsAg as detectable in patient blood.

4.2. Small-HBsAg

Inside the S-gene the different alleles a, d, y, w (four subdeterminants w1 to w4 are described), r and q can be distinguished [78]. The determinants d/y as well as w/r are mutually exclusive. This leads to at least 9 serotypes of the small-HBsAg. The a-determinant which is part of all HBs-subtypes can be divided into two alleles. They only differ in one amino acid (126 t = Thr, 126 i = Ile) [79]. The main subtypes are therefore designated ayw, ayr, adw and adr. Their geographical distribution was found to be stable over two decades. The subtype ayw was described in the Mediterranean countries (ayw2, ayw3), in West- and Central-Africa (ayw4, ayw2) and in Vietnam (ayw1). The rare subtype ayr is found in Vietnam. The subtype adw is predominant in North-West-Europe, in America, in East and South Africa, in India (adw2) and in South-East Asia (adw4). The subtype adr can be found in Polynesia (adrq-) and in South-East-Asia (adrq+) [80,81].

4.3. The Large-HBsAg and of the Medium-HBsAg

The medium-HBsAg (pre-S2) and the large-HBsAg (pre-S1) are very important for the virus clearence because they are more immunogenic and appear earlier in the course of infection than the small-HBsAg. Vaccines with all the three HBsAg were found to cause higher anti-HBs titers than vaccines with the small-HBsAg alone [85,86]. Recently, an A to G change at NT 2794 within the promotor of the large-HBsAg was found [83]. This mutation lead to a decreased protein expression and it may be speculated that immunological properties were altered. The pre-S1-region contains two important epitopes. One of them (aa 58 to 100) is speculated to be recognized by antibodies which are involved in viral clearance. The other one (aa 21 to 47) seems to be the hepatocyte binding region. A deletion of the antibody recognized region which does not touch the hepatocyte binding size could inhibit viral clearance [82, 84, 87, 88].

4.4. HBcAg and HBeAg

HBcAg and HBeAg are alternative translation products of the core gene, with HBeAg translation requiring an upstream precore region ATG codon (figure 2). The HBcAg (called "core protein" nowadays) assembles into viral nucleocapsid (core particle), which packages the pregenome (an RNA copy of viral DNA) and polymerase. Inside the core particle, the viral polymerase directs the synthesis of minus strand DNA from the RNA template. It then degrades the RNA pregenome and generates the plus strand DNA via the minus strand template.

The N-terminal 29 residues of the HBeAg precursor are specified by the precore region, the first 19 of which serve as the signal peptide to target the protein to the endoplasmic reticulum, where it is cleaved off. Further down the secretory pathway the argininerich C-terminus of the molecule is removed, thus releasing mature HBeAg into bloodstream. Therefore, HBeAg differs from core protein by a longer N-terminus and shorter C-terminal tail. However, thanks to an intramolecular disulfide bond HBeAg has a secondary structure quite different from that of core protein [91,94]. Only one of the two major B cell epitopes of HBeAg is shared with the core protein. HBeAg is not part of the virus particle, and its true function remains not fully understood. Expression of HBeAg is not required for virus replication in vitro [93]. Ablation of e antigen expression had no effect on the in vivo infectivity of the duck hepatitis B virus, but curtailed infection for the woodchuck hepatitis virus (which is more closely related to the human virus) [88 ,89, 92]. It was proposed that expression of HBeAg during perinatal infection, the major mode of HBV transmission in Asia, induces immune tolerance. Another potential role of HBeAg in promoting persistent infection is to mimic core protein so as to buffer immune attack of the infected hepatocytes by the anti-HBc antibodies. [90]

The translation within the C-gene can start at the precore start codon or at the start codon of the C region. If the ribosomes begin to translate at the precore start-codon they translate through the encapsidation signal. Thereby, a recognition of the hairpin structure is not possible and the growing polypeptide HBeAg is lead to the secretion pathway. If the translation starts at the start-codon of the Cregion, the encapsidation sequence is recognized and the developing HBcAg is encapsidated [95]. Various functional domains within the coreprotein could be distinguished. For the selfassembly of the virus capsid the 144 aa at the Nterminus of the core-protein are sufficient [96,97]. The arginine-rich C-terminus (up to aa 164) enables the encapsidation of the pregenomic RNA [97] and seems to stabilize the capsid by proteinnucleic acid interactions [96]. The remaining C-terminus (up to aa 173) may be important for the synthesis of plus-strand-DNA and thereby for the virus replication [97]. Furthermore the different epitopes within the core-protein differ in immunological aspects.

HBcAg and HBeAg are highly cross-reactive at the T-cell level [98,99]. It therefore may be speculated that HBeAg presents immunogenic epitopes to the T-cells thus protecting the HBcAg expressing hepatocytes against the immune system. After the selection of a HBeAg-negative mutant the epitopes of the HBcAg might come under the pressure of the immune system [100].

Antibody to HBsAg, produced in response to exposure to the envelope antigen, confers protective immunity. The antibody is detectable in patients who have recovered from acute hepatitis B and in those immunized with HBV vaccine, but it may become undetectable in patients who have recovered fully from infection. Antibody to HBcAg is detected in virtually all patients who have ever been exposed to HBV. Unlike antibody to HBsAg, this antibody is not protective; its presence alone cannot be used to distinguish acute from chronic infection. Patients who have persistent HBV infection are positive for antibody to HBcAg, as are those who have recovered from HBV infection. The IgM subtype of antibody to HBcAg is associated with acute infection and is therefore helpful in distinguishing acute from chronic infection. IgM antibody usually disappears within four to eight months after acute infection. Since some patients with chronic hepatitis B become positive for IgM antibody during flares in their disease, its presence is not an absolutely reliable marker of acute illness .[101] Antibody to

HBeAg appears once the antigen has been cleared and the virus is no longer replicating.

The presence of HBV DNA in serum, the best indication of active viral replication, can be detected by PCR-based technique. Studies have found HBV DNA level to be a strong predictor for the development of cirrhosis and HCC, irrespective of the status of viral and biochemical factors [102-108]. Some patients with HBsAg seroclearance have favorable biochemical, virologic, and histological parameters in the Chinese patients [109,110], but among patients who have seroconverted to antibody to HBsAg (anti-HBs) HCC due to HBV can occur [111]. Hepatitis B e antigen (HBeAg) is a biomarker of active viral proliferation in hepatocytes and infectivity. Among HBsAg carriers presenting HBeAg, HBV replication occurred more often and was more intensified than in HBsAg carriers presenting antibody to HBeAg (anti-HBe) [112]. A long-term follow-up study has shown a significantly elevated HCC risk for seropositives of both HBsAg and HBeAg compared with seropositives of HBsAg only and seronegatives [113]. Some results suggest that spontaneous HBeAg seroconversion confers favorable long-term outcomes. However, active hepatitis still may develop and lead to LC and HCC [114]. It was reported that two serum biomarkers such as $M(r)$ 7772 and 393 were identified by surface enhanced laser desorption/ionization time-of-flight (SELDI-TOF) mass spectrometry, which might be used for diagnosis and assessment of HBV-induced LC progression [115].

4.5. HBxAg

Previously, hepatitis B x antigen (HBxAg) has been shown to alter the expression of cellular genes that promote hepatocellular growth, survival, and tumorigenesis [116-120]. It is proposed that these proteins trigger corresponding antibody responses that may accompany the onset of critical transforming events. The antibody to HBxAg (anti-HBx) may serve as preneoplastic marker for HCC in HBV carriers with chronic liver disease, and may be identified by a simple blood test [121]. Study has given a full correlation between anti-HBx positivity in serum and HBxAg in HCC tissues [122,123]. HBx-dependent transformed phenotype is reversible by the expression of a single-chain variable fragment (scFv) specific to HBx, designated as H7scFv [124]. Thereby, HBx may be a good molecular target for the treatment of HBV-related tumors.

References

[1]   Ganem D, Prince AM.(2004).Hepatitis B virus infection--natural history and clinical consequences. *N. Engl. J. Med*, 350(11):1118-1129.

[2]   Tiollais P, Pourcel C, Dejean A.(1985)The hepatitis B virus. *Nature*, 317 (6037):489-495.

[3]   Santantonio T, Jung MC, Miska S, Pastore G, Pape GR, Will H.(1991).Prevalence and type of pre-C HBV mutants in anti-HBe positive carriers with chronic liver disease in a highly endemic area. *Virology*, 183(2):840-844

[4]   Hawkins AE, Gilson RJ, Bickerton EA, Tedder RS, Weller IV.(1994).Conservation of precore and core sequences of hepatitis B virus in chronic viral carriers. *J. Med. Virol*, 43(1):5-12.

[5]   Schödel F, Peterson D, Zheng J, Jones JE, Hughes JL, Milich DR. (1993). Structure of hepatitis B virus core and e-antigen .A single precore amino acid prevents nucleocapsid assembly. *J. Biol. Chem*, 268(2):1332-1337.

[6]   Takahashi K, Kishimoto S, Ohori K, Yoshizawa H, Machida A, Ohnuma H, Tsuda F, Munekata E, Miyakawa Y, Mayumi M. (1991).Molecular heterogeneity of e antigen polypeptides in sera from carriers of hepatitis B virus. *J. Immunol*, 147(9):3156-3160.

[7]   Persing DH, Varmus HE, Ganem D. (1986).Inhibition of secretion of hepatitis B surface antigen by a related presurface polypeptide. *Science*, 234(4782):1388-1391.

[8]   Neurath AR, Kent SB, Strick N, Parker K. (1986).Identification and chemical synthesis of a host cell receptor binding site on hepatitis B virus. *Cell*, 46(3):429-436

[9]   Milich DR, McLachlan A, Moriarty A, Thornton GB.(1987). A single 10-residue pre-S(1) peptide can prime T cell help for antibody production to multiple epitopes within the pre-S(1), pre-S(2), and S regions of HBsAg. *J. Immunol*, 138(12):4457-4465.

[10]   Milich DR, McLachlan A, Chisari FV, Kent SB, Thorton GB.(1986).Immune response to the Pre-S (1) region of the hepatitis B surface antigen (HBsAg): A Pre-S (1)-specific T cell response can bypass nonresponsiveness to the pre-S(2) and S regions of HBsAg. *J. Immunol*, 137: 315–322

[11]   Milich DR.(1987) Genetic and molecular basis for T- and B-cell recognition of hepatitis B viral antigens. *Immunol. Rev*, 99:71-103.

[12]   Jilg W.(1998).Novel hepatitis B vaccines. *Vaccine*, 16 Suppl: S65-S68.

[13]   Bartenschlager R, Schaller H.(1988).The amino-terminal domain of the hepadnaviral P-gene encodes the terminal protein (genome-linked protein) believed to prime reverse transcription. *Embo J*, 7(13):4185-4192.

[14]   Chang LJ, Hirsch RC, Ganem D, Varmus HE. (1990). Effects of insertional and point mutations on the functions of the duck hepatitis B virus polymerase. *J. Virol*, 64(11):5553-5558.

[15]   Radziwill G, Tucker W, Schaller H. (1990).Mutational analysis of the hepatitis B virus P gene product: domain structure and RNase H activity. *J. Virol*, 64(2):613-620.

[16]   Lanford RE, Notvall L, Beames B.(1995).Nucleotide priming and reverse transcriptase activity of hepatitis B virus polymerase expressed in insect cells. *J. Virol*, 69(7):4431-4439.

[17]   Saldanha JA, Qiu H, Thomas HC, Monjardino J. (1992). Mapping of 5' ends of virion-derived HBV DNA. *Virology*, 188(1):358-361.

[18]   Gerlich WH, Robinson WS. (1980).Hepatitis B virus contains protein attached to the 5' terminus of its complete DNA strand. *Cell*, 21(3):801-809.

[19]   Zoulim F, Seeger C.(1994).Reverse transcription in hepatitis B viruses is primed by a tyrosine residue of the polymerase. *J. Virol*, 68(1):6-13.

[20]   Wang GH, Seeger C. (1993).Novel mechanism for reverse transcription in hepatitis B viruses. *J. Virol*, 67(11):6507-6512.

[21]   Kumar V, Jayasuryan N, Kumar R. (1996).A truncated mutant (residues 58-140) of the hepatitis B virus X protein retains transactivation function. *Proc. Natl. Acad. Sci. USA*, 93(11):5647-5652.

[22]   Murakami S, Cheong JH, Kaneko S. (1994). Human hepatitis virus X gene encodes a regulatory domain that represses transactivation of X protein. *J. Biol. Chem*, 269(21):15118-15123.

[23]   Faktor O, Shaul Y. (1990). The identification of hepatitis B virus X gene responsive elements reveals functional similarity of X and HTLV-I tax. *Oncogene*, 5 (6):867-872.

[24]   Seto E, Mitchell PJ, Yen TS. (1990). Transactivation by the hepatitis B virus X protein depends on AP-2 and other transcription factors. *Nature*, 344(6261):72-74.

[25]   Wu JY, Zhou ZY, Judd A, Cartwright CA, Robinson WS.(1990). The hepatitis B virus-encoded transcriptional trans-activator hbx appears to be a novel protein serine/threonine kinase. *Cell*, 63(4):687-695.

[26]   Norder H, Courouce AM, Magnius LO. (1993).Complete nucleotide
        sequences of six hepatitis B viral genomes encoding the surface antigen
        subtypes ayw4, adw4q-, and adrq- and their phylogenetic classification.
        Arch. Virol. Suppl, 8:189-199.

[27]   Norder H, Courouce AM, Magnius LO.(1994).Complete genomes,
        phylogenetic relatedness, and structural proteins of six strains of the
        hepatitis B virus, four of which represent two new genotypes. *Virology*,
        198(2):489-503.

[28]   Norder H, Hammas B, Lofdahl S, Courouce AM, Magnius LO.
        (1992).Comparison of the amino acid sequences of nine different
        serotypes of hepatitis B surface antigen and genomic classification of the
        corresponding hepatitis B virus strains. *J. Gen. Virol*, 73(Pt 5):1201-1208.

[29]   Okamoto H, Tsuda F, Sakugawa H, Sastrosoewignjo RI, Imai M,
        Miyakawa Y, Mayumi M.(1988).Typing hepatitis B virus by homology in
        nucleotide sequence: comparison of surface antigen subtypes. *J. Gen.
        Virol*, 69 (Pt 10):2575-2583.

[30]   Kao JH. (2002). Hepatitis B viral genotypes: clinical relevance and
        molecular characteristics. *J. Gastroenterol. Hepatol*, 17(6):643-650.

[31]   Naumann H, Schaefer S, Yoshida CF, Gaspar AM, Repp R, Gerlich WH.
        (1993). Identification of a new hepatitis B virus (HBV) genotype from
        Brazil that expresses HBV surface antigen subtype adw4. *J. Gen. Virol*,
        74 (Pt 8):1627-1632.

[32]   Stuyver L, De Gendt S, Van Geyt C, Zoulim F, Fried M, Schinazi RF,
        Rossau R. (2000). A new genotype of hepatitis B virus: complete genome
        and phylogenetic relatedness. *J. Gen. Virol*, 81(Pt 1):67-74.

[33]   Arauz-Ruiz P, Norder H, Robertson BH, Magnius LO. (2002). Genotype
        H: a new Amerindian genotype of hepatitis B virus revealed in Central
        America. *J. Gen. Virol*, 83(Pt 8):2059-2073.

[34]   Chu CJ, Keeffe EB, Han SH, Perrillo RP, Min AD, Soldevila-Pico C,
        Carey W, Brown RS, Jr., Luketic VA, Terrault N, Lok AS.(2003).
        Hepatitis B virus genotypes in the United States: results of a nationwide
        study. *Gastroenterology*, 125(2):444-451.

[35]   Chu CJ, Lok AS.(2002).Clinical significance of hepatitis B virus
        genotypes. *Hepatology*, 35(5):1274-1276.

[36] Blitz L, Pujol FH, Swenson PD, Porto L, Atencio R, Araujo M, Costa L, Monsalve DC, Torres JR, Fields HA, Lambert S, Van Geyt C, Norder H, Magnius LO, Echevarria JM, Stuyver L. (1998). Antigenic diversity of hepatitis B virus strains of genotype F in Amerindians and other population groups from Venezuela. *J. Clin. Microbiol*, 36(3):648-651.

[37] Mbayed VA, Lopez JL, Telenta PF, Palacios G, Badia I, Ferro A, Galoppo C, Campos R.(1998).Distribution of hepatitis B virus genotypes in two different pediatric populations from Argentina. *J. Clin. Microbiol*, 36(11):3362-3365.

[38] Telenta PF, Poggio GP, Lopez JL, Gonzalez J, Lemberg A, Campos RH.(1997). Increased prevalence of genotype F hepatitis B virus isolates in Buenos Aires, Argentina. *J. Clin. Microbiol*, 35(7):1873-1875.

[39] Mayerat C, Mantegani A, Frei PC.(1999). Does hepatitis B virus (HBV) genotype influence the clinical outcome of HBV infection? *J. Viral. Hepat*, 6(4):299-304.

[40] Sugauchi F, Orito E, Ichida T, Kato H, Sakugawa H, Kakumu S, Ishida T, Chutaputti A, Lai CL, Ueda R, Miyakawa Y, Mizokami M. (2002).Hepatitis B virus of genotype B with or without recombination with genotype C over the precore region plus the core gene. *J. Virol*, 76(12):5985-5992.

[41] Sugauchi F, Mizokami M, Orito E, Ohno T, Kato H, Suzuki S, Kimura Y, Ueda R, Butterworth LA, Cooksley WG. (2001).A novel variant genotype C of hepatitis B virus identified in isolates from Australian Aborigines: complete genome sequence and phylogenetic relatedness. *J. Gen. Virol*, 82(Pt 4):883-892.

[42] Kramvis A, Weitzmann L, Owiredu WK, Kew MC. (2002). Analysis of the complete genome of subgroup A' hepatitis B virus isolates from South Africa. *J. Gen. Virol*, 83(Pt 4):835-839.

[43] Sugauchi F, Orito E, Ichida T, Kato H, Sakugawa H, Kakumu S, Ishida T, Chutaputti A, Lai CL, Gish RG, Ueda R, Miyakawa Y, Mizokami M. (2003).Epidemiologic and virologic characteristics of hepatitis B virus genotype B having the recombination with genotype C. *Gastroenterology*, 124(4):925-932.

[44] Norder H, Arauz-Ruiz P, Blitz L, Pujol FH, Echevarria JM, Magnius LO. (2003). The T(1858) variant predisposing to the precore stop mutation correlates with one of two major genotype F hepatitis B virus clades. *J. Gen. Virol*, 84(Pt 8):2083-2087.

[45]   Norder H, Courouce AM, Coursaget P, Echevarria JM, Lee SD, Mushahwar IK, Robertson BH, Locarnini S, Magnius LO. (2004).Genetic diversity of hepatitis B virus strains derived worldwide: genotypes, subgenotypes, and HBsAg subtypes. *Intervirology*, 47(6):289-309.

[46]   Shiina S, Fujino H, Uta Y, Tagawa K, Unuma T, Yoneyama M, Ohmori T, Suzuki S, Kurita M, Ohashi Y.(1991). Relationship of HBsAg subtypes with HBeAg/anti-HBe status and chronic liver disease. Part I: Analysis of 1744 HBsAg carriers. *Am. J. Gastroenterol*, 86(7):866-871.

[47]   Lindh M, Hannoun C, Dhillon AP, Norkrans G, Horal P.(1999).Core promoter mutations and genotypes in relation to viral replication and liver damage in East Asian hepatitis B virus carriers. *J. Infect. Dis*, 179(4):775-782.

[48]   Kao JH, Chen PJ, Lai MY, Chen DS.(2000). Hepatitis B genotypes correlate with clinical outcomes in patients with chronic hepatitis B. *Gastroenterology*, 118(3):554-559.

[49]   Sumi H, Yokosuka O, Seki N, Arai M, Imazeki F, Kurihara T, Kanda T, Fukai K, Kato M, Saisho H.(2003). Influence of hepatitis B virus genotypes on the progression of chronic type B liver disease. *Hepatology*, 37(1):19-26.

[50]   Orito E, Mizokami M, Sakugawa H, Michitaka K, Ishikawa K, Ichida T, Okanoue T, Yotsuyanagi H, Iino S. (2001).A case-control study for clinical and molecular biological differences between hepatitis B viruses of genotypes B and C. *Hepatology*, 33(1):218-223.

[51]   Chu CJ, Hussain M, Lok AS.(2002).Hepatitis B virus genotype B is associated with earlier HBeAg seroconversion compared with hepatitis B virus genotype C. *Gastroenterology*, 122(7):1756-1762.

[52]   Ding X, Mizokami M, Yao G, Xu B, Orito E, Ueda R, Nakanishi M. (2001).Hepatitis B virus genotype distribution among chronic hepatitis B virus carriers in Shanghai, China. *Intervirology*, 44(1):43-47.

[53]   Sanchez-Tapias JM, Costa J, Mas A, Bruguera M, Rodes J. (2002). Influence of hepatitis B virus genotype on the long-term outcome of chronic hepatitis B in western patients. *Gastroenterology*, 123(6):1848-1856.

[54]   Imamura T, Yokosuka O, Kurihara T, Kanda T, Fukai K, Imazeki F, Saisho H. (2003).Distribution of hepatitis B viral genotypes and mutations in the core promoter and precore regions in acute forms of liver disease in patients from Chiba, Japan. *Gut*, 52(11):1630-1637.

[55]   Kao JH, Chen PJ, Lai MY, Chen DS.(2000).Hepatitis B genotypes correlate with clinical outcomes in patients with chronic hepatitis B. *Gastroente-rology.* 118(3):554–9.

[56]   Chu, CJ, Hussain, M. and Lok, AS. (2002). Hepatitis B virus genotype B is associated with earlier HBeAg seroconversion compared with hepatitis B virus genotype C. *Gastroenterology.* 122:1756–62.

[57]   Nakayoshi T, Maeshiro T, Nakayoshi T, Nakasone H, Sakugawa H, Kinjo F, Orito E, Mizokami M. (2003). Difference in prognosis between patients infected with hepatitis B virus with genotype B and those with genotype C in the Okinawa Islands: a prospective study. *J. Med. Virol,* 70(3):350-354.

[58]   Tsubota A, Arase Y, Ren F, Tanaka H, Ikeda K, Kumada H. (2001). Genotype may correlate with liver carcinogenesis and tumor characteristics in cirrhotic patients infected with hepatitis B virus subtype adw. *J. Med. Virol,* 65(2):257-265.

[59]   Fujie H, Moriya K, Shintani Y, Yotsuyanagi H, Iino S, Koike K. (2001).Hepatitis B virus genotypes and hepatocellular carcinoma in Japan. *Gastroenterology,* 120(6):1564-1565.

[60]   Lee CM, Chen CH, Lu SN, Tung HD, Chou WJ, Wang JH, Chen TM, Hung CH, Huang CC, Chen WJ.(2003).Prevalence and clinical implications of hepatitis B virus genotypes in southern Taiwan. *Scand. J. Gastroenterol,* 38(1):95-101.

[61]   Duong TN, Horiike N, Michitaka K, Yan C, Mizokami M, Tanaka Y, Jyoko K, Yamamoto K, Miyaoka H, Yamashita Y, Ohno N, Onji M. Comparison of genotypes C and D of the hepatitis B virus in Japan: a clinical and molecular biological study. *J. Med. Virol,* 2004, 72(4):551-557

[62]   Thakur V, Guptan RC, Kazim SN, Malhotra V, Sarin SK. (2002).Profile, spectrum and significance of HBV genotypes in chronic liver disease patients in the Indian subcontinent. *J. Gastroenterol. Hepatol,* 17(2):165-170.

[63]   Dooley JS, Davis GL, Peters M, Waggoner JG, Goodman Z, Hoofnagle JH.(1986).Pilot study of recombinant human alpha-interferon for chronic type B hepatitis. *Gastroenterology,* 90(1):150-157.

[64]   Hoofnagle JH, Peters M, Mullen KD, Jones DB, Rustgi V, Di Bisceglie A, Hallahan C, Park Y, Meschievitz C, Jones EA. (1988). Randomized, controlled trial of recombinant human alpha-interferon in patients with chronic hepatitis B. *Gastroenterology,* 95(5):1318-1325.

[65] Wong DK, Cheung AM, O'Rourke K, Naylor CD, Detsky AS, Heathcote J. (1993).Effect of alpha-interferon treatment in patients with hepatitis B e antigen-positive chronic hepatitis B.A meta-analysis. *Ann. Intern. Med*, 119(4):312-323.

[66] Zhang X, Zoulim F, Habersetzer F, Xiong S, Trepo C.(1996).Analysis of hepatitis B virus genotypes and pre-core region variability during interferon treatment of HBe antigen negative chronic hepatitis B. *J. Med. Virol*, 48(1):8-16.

[67] Kao JH, Wu NH, Chen PJ, Lai MY, Chen DS.(2000).Hepatitis B genotypes and the response to interferon therapy. *J. Hepatol*, 33(6):998-1002.

[68] Wai CT, Chu CJ, Hussain M, Lok AS.(2002). HBV genotype B is associated with better response to interferon therapy in HBeAg(+) chronic hepatitis than genotype C. *Hepatology*, 36(6):1425-1430.

[69] Nevens F, Main J, Honkoop P, Tyrrell DL, Barber J, Sullivan MT, Fevery J, De Man RA, Thomas HC. (1997). Lamivudine therapy for chronic hepatitis B: a six-month randomized dose-ranging study. *Gastroenterology*, 113(4):1258-1263.

[70] Lai CL, Ching CK, Tung AK, Li E, Young J, Hill A, Wong BC, Dent J, Wu PC. (1997). Lamivudine is effective in suppressing hepatitis B virus DNA in Chinese hepatitis B surface antigen carriers: a placebo-controlled trial. *Hepatology*, 25(1):241-244.

[71] Suzuki Y, Kumada H, Ikeda K, Chayama K, Arase Y, Saitoh S, Tsubota A, Kobayashi M, Koike M, Ogawa N, Tanikawa K.(1999). Histological changes in liver biopsies after one year of lamivudine treatment in patients with chronic hepatitis B infection. *J. Hepatol*, 30(5):743-748.

[72] Dienstag JL, Schiff ER, Wright TL, Perrillo RP, Hann HW, Goodman Z, Crowther L, Condreay LD, Woessner M, Rubin M, Brown NA.(1999).Lamivudine as initial treatment for chronic hepatitis B in the United States. *N. Engl. J. Med*, 341(17):1256-1263.

[73] Liaw YF, Leung NW, Chang TT, Guan R, Tai DI, Ng KY, Chien RN, Dent J, Roman L, Edmundson S, Lai CL. (2000).Effects of extended lamivudine therapy in Asian patients with chronic hepatitis B. Asia Hepatitis Lamivudine Study Group. *Gastroenterology*, 119(1):172-180.

[74] Chien RN, Yeh CT, Tsai SL, Chu CM, Liaw YF.(2003).Determinants for sustained HBeAg response to lamivudine therapy. *Hepatology*,38(5):1267-1273.

[75]   Qaqish RB, Mattes KA, Ritchie DJ. (2003). Adefovir dipivoxil: a new antiviral agent for the treatment of hepatitis B virus infection. *Clin. Ther*, 25(12):3084-3099.

[76]   Angus P, Vaughan R, Xiong S, Yang H, Delaney W, Gibbs C, Brosgart C, Colledge D, Edwards R, Ayres A, Bartholomeusz A, Locarnini S. (2003). Resistance to adefovir dipivoxil therapy associated with the selection of a novel mutation in the HBV polymerase. *Gastroenterology*, 125(2):292-297.

[77]   Westland C, Delaney Wt, Yang H, Chen SS, Marcellin P, Hadziyannis S, Gish R, Fry J, Brosgart C, Gibbs C, Miller M, Xiong S.(2003). Hepatitis B virus genotypes and virologic response in 694 patients in phase III studies of adefovir dipivoxil1. *Gastroenterology*, 125(1):107-116.

[78]   Norder H, Courouce AM, Magnius LO.(1992).Molecular basis of hepatitis B virus serotype variations within the four major subtypes. *J. Gen. Virol*, 73 (Pt 12):3141-3145.

[79]   Ohnuma H, Machida A, Okamoto H, Tsuda F, Sakamoto M, Tanaka T, Miyakawa Y, Mayumi M.(1993).Allelic subtypic determinants of hepatitis B surface antigen (i and t) that are distinct from d/y or w/r. *J. Virol*, 67(2):927-932.

[80]   Kidd-Ljunggren K.(1996). Variability in hepatitis B virus DNA: phylogenetic, epidemiological and clinical implications. *Scand. J. Infect. Dis*, 28(2):111-116.

[81]   Courouce-Pauty AM, Plancon A, Soulier JP. (1983). Distribution of HBsAg subtypes in the world. *Vox Sang*, 44(4):197-211.

[82]   Fiordalisi G, Ghiotto F, Castelnuovo F, Primi D, Cariani E.(1994).Analysis of the hepatitis B virus genome and immune response in HBsAg, anti-HBs positive chronic hepatitis. *J. Hepatol*, 20(4):487-493.

[83]   Schories M, Peters T, Rasenack J.(2000).Isolation, characterization and biological significance of hepatitis B virus mutants from serum of a patient with immunologically negative HBV infection. *J. Hepatol*, 33(5):799-811.

[84]   Yamamoto K, Horikita M, Tsuda F, Itoh K, Akahane Y, Yotsumoto S, Okamoto H, Miyakawa Y, Mayumi M.(1994).Naturally occurring escape mutants of hepatitis B virus with various mutations in the S gene in carriers seropositive for antibody to hepatitis B surface antigen. *J. Virol*, 68(4):2671-2676.

[85] Yap I, Chan SH.(1996). A new pre-S containing recombinant hepatitis B vaccine and its effect on non-responders: a preliminary observation. *Ann. Acad. Med. Singapore,* 25(1):120-122.

[86] Yap I, Guan R, Chan SH. (1995).Study on the comparative immunogenicity of a recombinant DNA hepatitis B vaccine containing pre-S components of the HBV coat protein with non pre-S containing vaccines. *J. Gastroenterol. Hepatol,* 10(1):51-55.

[87] Fernholz D, Galle PR, Stemler M, Brunetto M, Bonino F, Will H.(1993).Infectious hepatitis B virus variant defective in pre-S2 protein expression in a chronic carrier. *Virology,* 194(1):137-148.

[88] Chang C, Enders G, Sprengel R, Peters N, Varmus HE, Ganem D.(1987). Expression of the precore region of an avian hepatitis B virus is not required for viral replication. *J. Virol,* 61(10):3322-3325.

[89] Chen HS, Kew MC, Hornbuckle WE, Tennant BC, Cote PJ, Gerin JL, Purcell RH, Miller RH. (1992).The precore gene of the woodchuck hepatitis virus genome is not essential for viral replication in the natural host. *J. Virol,* 66(9):5682-5684.

[90] Milich D, Liang TJ. (2003). Exploring the biological basis of hepatitis B e antigen in hepatitis B virus infection. *Hepatology,* 38(5):1075-1086.

[91] Nassal M, Rieger A. (1993). An intramolecular disulfide bridge between Cys-7 and Cys61 determines the structure of the secretory core gene product (e antigen) of hepatitis B virus. *J. Virol,* 67(7):4307-4315.

[92] Schlicht HJ, Salfeld J, Schaller H.(1987).The duck hepatitis B virus pre-C region encodes a signal sequence which is essential for synthesis and secretion of processed core proteins but not for virus formation. *J. Virol,* 61(12):3701-3709.

[93] Tong SP, Diot C, Gripon P, Li J, Vitvitski L, Trepo C, Guguen-Guillouzo C. (1991).In vitro replication competence of a cloned hepatitis B virus variant with a nonsense mutation in the distal pre-C region. *Virology,* 181(2):733-737.

[94] Wasenauer G, Kock J, Schlicht HJ.(1993).Relevance of cysteine residues for biosynthesis and antigenicity of human hepatitis B virus e protein. *J. Virol,* 67(3):1315-1321.

[95] Nassal M, Junker-Niepmann M, Schaller H. (1990). Translational inactivation of RNA function: discrimination against a subset of genomic transcripts during HBV nucleocapsid assembly. *Cell,* 63(6):1357-1363.

[96]   Birnbaum F, Nassal M. (1990). Hepatitis B virus nucleocapsid assembly: primary structure requirements in the core protein. *J. Virol*, 64(7):3319-3330.

[97]   Nassal M. (1992). The arginine-rich domain of the hepatitis B virus core protein is required for pregenome encapsidation and productive viral positive-strand DNA synthesis but not for virus assembly. *J. Virol*, 66(7):4107-4116.

[98]   Milich DR, McLachlan A, Moriarty A, Thornton GB.(1987).Immune response to hepatitis B virus core antigen (HBcAg): localization of T cell recognition sites within HBcAg/HBeAg. *J. Immunol*, 4: 1223–1231.

[99]   Milich DR, McLachlan A, Stahl S, Wingfield P, Thornton GB, Hughes JL, Jones JE.(1988).Comparative immunogenicity of hepatitis B virus core and E antigen. *J. Immunol*, 141(10):3617-3624.

[100]   Carman W, Thomas H, Domingo E. (1993).Viral genetic variation: hepatitis B virus as a clinical example. *Lancet*, 341(8841):349-353.

[101]   Milich DR, Sallberg M, Maruyama T. (1995).The humoral immune response in acute and chronic hepatitis B virus infection. *Springer Semin. Immunopathol*, 17(2-3):149-166.

[102]   Jun EJ, Han JY, Choi H, Chang UI, Lee TK, Kim YH, Kim JI, Park SH, Kim JK, Chung KW, Sun HS.(2002). The clinical significance of quantitation of HBV DNA in serum-comparison of the branched-DNA assay with the second-generation digene hybrid capture assay and long-term observation. *Taehan Kan Hakhoe Chi*, 8(2):157-166.

[103]   Ikeda K, Arase Y, Kobayashi M, Someya T, Saitoh S, Suzuki Y, Suzuki F, Tsubota A, Akuta N, Kumada H.(2003).Consistently low hepatitis B virus DNA saves patients from hepatocellular carcinogenesis in HBV-related cirrhosis.A nested case-control study using 96 untreated patients. *Intervirology*, 46(2):96-104.

[104]   Shimada S, Aizawa R, Abe H, Suto S, Miyakawa Y, Aizawa Y. (2003). Analysis of risk factors for hepatocellular carcinoma that is negative for hepatitis B surface antigen (HBsAg). *Intern. Med*, 42(5):389-393.

[105]   Ohata K, Hamasaki K, Toriyama K, Ishikawa H, Nakao K, Eguchi K.(2004). High viral load is a risk factor for hepatocellular carcinoma in patients with chronic hepatitis B virus infection. *J. Gastroenterol. Hepatol*, 19(6):670-675.

[106] Ikeda K, Kobayashi M, Saitoh S, Someya T, Hosaka T, Akuta N, Suzuki Y, Suzuki F, Tsubota A, Arase Y, Kumada H.(2005). Significance of hepatitis B virus DNA clearance and early prediction of hepatocellular carcinogenesis in patients with cirrhosis undergoing interferon therapy: long-term follow up of a pilot study. *J. Gastroenterol. Hepatol*, 20(1):95-102.

[107] Liaw YF.(2005).Prevention and surveillance of hepatitis B virus-related hepatocellular carcinoma. *Semin. Liver Dis* , 25 Suppl 1:40-47.

[108] Mahmood S, Niiyama G, Kamei A, Izumi A, Nakata K, Ikeda H, Suehiro M, Kawanaka M, Togawa K, Yamada G. (2005). Influence of viral load and genotype in the progression of Hepatitis B-associated liver cirrhosis to hepatocellular carcinoma. *Liver Int*, 25(2):220-225.

[109] Yuen MF, Wong DK, Sablon E, Tse E, Ng IO, Yuan HJ, Siu CW, Sander TJ, Bourne EJ, Hall JG, Condreay LD, Lai CL. (2004). HBsAg seroclearance in chronic hepatitis B in the Chinese: virological, histological, and clinical aspects. *Hepatology*, 39(6):1694-1701.

[110] Ahn SH, Park YN, Park JY, Chang HY, Lee JM, Shin JE, Han KH, Park C, Moon YM, Chon CY. (2005).Long-term clinical and histological outcomes in patients with spontaneous hepatitis B surface antigen seroclearance. *J. Hepatol*, 42(2):188-194.

[111] Tsuboi Y, Ohkoshi S, Yano M, Suzuki K, Tsubata SS, Ishihara K, Ichida T, Sugitani S, Shibazaki K, Aoyagi Y. (2006). Common clinicopathological features of the patients with chronic hepatitis B virus infection who developed hepatocellular carcinoma after seroconversion to anti-HBs--a consideration of the pathogenesis of HBV-induced hepatocellular carcinoma and a strategy to inhibit it. *Hepatogastroenterology*, 53(67):110-114.

[112] Lapinski TW, Kowalczuk O, Prokopowicz D, Chyczewski L, Jaroszewicz J. (2005).HBV-DNA and sFas, sFasL concentrations in serum of healthy HBsAg carriers. *Rocz. Akad. Med. Bialymst*, 50:179-182.

[113] You SL, Yang HI, Chen CJ.(2004).Seropositivity of hepatitis B e antigen and hepatocellular carcinoma. *Ann. Med*, 36(3):215-224.

[114] Hsu YS, Chien RN, Yeh CT, Sheen IS, Chiou HY, Chu CM, Liaw YF. (2002). Long-term outcome after spontaneous HBeAg seroconversion in patients with chronic hepatitis B. *Hepatology*,35(6):1522-1527.

[115] Zhu XD, Zhang WH, Li CL, Xu Y, Liang WJ, Tien P.(2004).New serum biomarkers for detection of HBV-induced liver cirrhosis using SELDI protein chip technology. *World J. Gastroenterol*, 10(16):2327-2329.

[116] Lian Z, Pan J, Liu J, Zhang S, Zhu M, Arbuthnot P, Kew M, Feitelson MA. (1999).The translation initiation factor, hu-Sui1 may be a target of hepatitis B X antigen in hepatocarcinogenesis. *Oncogene*, 18(9):1677-1687.

[117] Lian Z, Liu J, Pan J, Satiroglu Tufan NL, Zhu M, Arbuthnot P, Kew M, Clayton MM, Feitelson MA. (2001). A cellular gene up-regulated by hepatitis B virus-encoded X antigen promotes hepatocellular growth and survival. *Hepatology*, 34(1):146-157.

[118] Tufan NL, Lian Z, Liu J, Pan J, Arbuthnot P, Kew M, Clayton MM, Zhu M, Feitelson MA. (2002). Hepatitis B x antigen stimulates expression of a novel cellular gene, URG4, that promotes hepatocellular growth and survival. *Neoplasia*, 4(4):355-368.

[119] Lian Z, Liu J, Li L, Li X, Tufan NL, Clayton M, Wu MC, Wang HY, Arbuthnot P, Kew M, Feitelson MA.(2003).Upregulated expression of a unique gene by hepatitis B x antigen promotes hepatocellular growth and tumorigenesis. *Neoplasia*, 5(3):229-244.

[120] Lian Z, Liu J, Li L, Li X, Tufan NL, Wu MC, Wang HY, Arbuthnot P, Kew M, Feitelson MA. (2004).Human S15a expression is upregulated by hepatitis B virus X protein. *Mol. Carcinog*, 40(1):34-46.

[121] Hann HW, Lee J, Bussard A, Liu C, Jin YR, Guha K, Clayton MM, Ardlie K, Pellini MJ, Feitelson MA.(2004).Preneoplastic markers of hepatitis B virus-associated hepatocellular carcinoma. *Cancer Res*, 64(20):7329-7335.

[122] Lopez JB.(2005).Recent developments in the first detection of hepatocellular carcinoma. *Clin. Biochem. Rev*, 26(3):65-79.

[123] Hwang GY, Lin CY, Huang LM, Wang YH, Wang JC, Hsu CT, Yang SS, Wu CC. (2003).Detection of the hepatitis B virus X protein (HBx) antigen and anti-HBx antibodies in cases of human hepatocellular carcinoma. *J. Clin. Microbiol*, 41(12):5598-5603.

[124] Jin YH, Kwon MH, Kim K, Shin HJ, Shin JS, Cho H, Park S. (2006). An intracellular antibody can suppress tumorigenicity in hepatitis B virus X-expressing cells. *Cancer Immunol. Immunother*, 55(5):569-578.

Chapter III

Immunopathogenesis of HBV Infection

I. Natural History, Life Cycle, Mutation, and Coinfection

Viral hepatitis is a necroinflammatory liver disease of variable severity. Most studies suggest that the hepatitis viruses are not directly cytopathic, or at least not highly cytopathic, for the infected hepatocytes. Indeed, based on fairly extensive studies of HBV pathogenesis in man and animal models, there is considerable evidence that viral hepatitis is initiated by an antigen-specific antiviral cellular immune response. Some data also suggest that noncytolytic intracellular viral inactivation by certain inflammatory cytokines released from activated lymphomononuclear cells may play an important role in the clearance of at least some of these viruses from the infected cells [1]. This appears to be true for HBV.

1. Natural History

Despite the presence of hepatitis B vaccine, new HBV infection remains common. Infection with HBV can result in both acute and chronic hepatitis. Acute infection develops after a 2- to 6-week incubation period when symptomatic hepatitis occurs and there is a subsequent resolution of liver enzymes. Hepatitis B surface antigen (HBsAg) is cleared after several months, but virus persists for life. Acute hepatitis is ordinarily a self-limited disease that includes flu-like symptoms, fever, joint pains, malaise, severe loss of appetite, and, in time, jaundice. Most patients recover in several weeks or months with no further symptoms, but a small percentage may develop fulminant hepatitis, which has a high mortality rate.

About 10% of patients with acute hepatitis will retain the infection and develop chronic hepatitis. Chronic disease is characterized by immune tolerance, with high HBV viral loads and the presence of hepatitis B e antigen (HBeAg). [2] Tolerance can last for decades, sometimes followed by immune competence. Immune responsiveness in HBV-infected patients leads to necroinflammatory disease, characterized by altered histology and biochemical and serologic markers. People with subclinical persistent infection, normal serum aminotransferase levels, and normal or nearly normal findings on liver biopsy are termed asymptomatic chronic HBV carrier, those with abnormal liver function and histological features are classified as having chronic hepatitis B [3].

In fact, chronic HBV infection presents as one of four potentially successive phases (figure 1). For its classification, serum aminotransferase ALT and quantitative HBVDNA in addition to HBeAg status are required. In the immunotolerant phase, serum HBeAg is detectable; serum HBV-DNA levels are high; and serum aminotransferases normal or minimally elevated. In the immunoactive phase, serum HBV DNA levels decrease and flares of aminotransferases may be observed. Over a period of months to years, these events are followed by HBeAg-anti-HBe seroconversion. The immune control phase follows HBeAg-anti-HBe seroconversion. HBV replication persists but at very low levels. This phase is usually termed the "inactive carrier state." In some patients, HBeAg seroconversion is accompanied by the selection of HBV variants that are unable to produce HBeAg. [4] A proportion of these HBeAg-negative patients may subsequently develop viral and liver disease reactivation, enter the immune escape phase, and progress to HBeAg-negative chronic hepatitis B. HBeAg-negative chronic hepatitis B is generally associated with a more severe liver disease with a very low rate of spontaneous disease remission and a low sustained response rate to antiviral therapy [5].

About 2% to 10% of those patients with chronic HBV will progress to compensated cirrhosis, 3% to 5% of whom will eventually experience decompensated disease and potentially progress to HCC or death. (figure 1) [6] Cirrhosis may develop as a consequence of repeated immune system attacks. Once established, cirrhosis cannot be cured; however, its progress may be stopped if the cause (in this case, HBV infection) is removed. Without treatment, the typical progression is from compensated cirrhosis to decompensated cirrhosis.

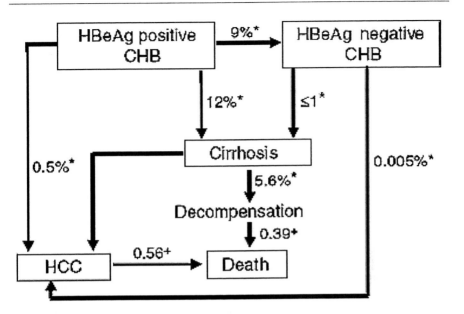

* Annual probability of variable
+Annual excess mortality rates

Figure 3.1. Natural course of chronic hepatitis B. HBeAg, hepatitis B e antigen; CHB, chronic hepatitis B; HCC, hepatocellular carcinoma.

The mortality rate at 5 years is 16% for those with compensated cirrhosis and is 65% to 86% for decompensated cirrhosis [7,8]. Genotype C is associated with a higher risk of cirrhosis than genotype B based on studies in Asian patients [9]. The decompensated cirrhosis is characterized by cessation of enzymatic processes in the liver and subsequent severe clinical complications such as fluid retention in the abdomen (ascites), jaundice, internal bleeding, and hepatic encephalopathy. Patients with decompensated cirrhosis are candidates for liver transplantation, without which death results from end-stage liver disease. In patients with compensated HBV cirrhosis, active viral replication correlates significantly with the risk of hepatic flare, decompensation, and the development of HCC [10].

2. Life Cycle

2.1. The Early Steps

In general, the early step of virus infection in which the virus enters the cell can be divided into three stages: attachment, fusion, and entry. The attachment usually is via the interaction of viral surface protein with the specific receptor on the cell membrane. However, the fusion of a viral envelope and cell membrane and the following viral genome release finally trigger the viral infection [11, 12].

The Attachment of HBV

The HBV surface protein antigens (HBsAg) are comprised of three carboxyl-co-terminal HBs proteins termed large (LHBs), middle (MHBs) and small (SHBs, also called major) protein [13,14]. LHBs is essential for attachment. The putative attachment site of HBV located in the amino acids 21–47 of preS1. [15-18] However, MHBs are probably also involved in viral entry. SHBs, the most abundant viral glycoprotein, certainly has a role in virus secretion [17, 18]. The limited availability of primary human tissue almost certainly hampers progress. Using human hepatoma cell line or the membrane of human liver cells, the protein that bind HBV MHBs or SHBs has been reported by several groups [19-22].

The HBV Fusion and Proteolysis

The attachment of HBV surface protein to the host cell is essential for HBV entry. However, attachment alone is not sufficient for viral infection. Attachment and fusion are two distinct events. Attachment usually is receptor mediated, and therefore, is highly cell specific. In contrast, viral fusion is dependent on a specific domain within the viral surface protein, known as the "fusion motif," which is normally composed of a series of hydrophobic amino acids [23-25]

Internalization of HBV Following Attachment

There are two entryways that the viruses use for their entry. One is via direct fusion with the host cell membrane like HIV [26] and the other is via endocytic pathway like Semliki forest virus and Influenza virus [12, 27]. Some data suggests that DHBV may use the endocytosis way for its entry [28]. This hypothesis was supported by the observation of the conformation change of the large surface protein of DHBV at low pH condition [29].

2.2. Life Cycle

After entry and presumptive uncoating (figure 3), viral plus strand DNA synthesis is completed and the nucleocapsid particle delivers the viral genome to the nucleus, where covalently closed circular (ccc) DNA molecule is yielded. HBV replication involves reverse transcription of the RNA pregenome to produce minus strand DNA. The minus strands then serve as the template for viral plus strand DNA synthesis, resulting in an encapsidated double-stranded open circular DNA genome that either recycles back to the nucleus to amplify the pool of cccDNA or becomes enveloped by the viral envelope proteins, buds into the endoplasmic reticulum (ER), and is secreted via the Golgi apparatus into the blood, where it can spread to other hepatocytes. The nascent precore protein contains the entire core protein plus a leader sequence that directs it to the ER, where it undergoes limited proteolysis and is secreted into the plasma as HBeAg. The envelope proteins are cotranslationally inserted into the ER membrane where they aggregate, bud into the ER lumen, and are secreted by the cell, either as subviral envelope particles or as infectious virions if they have enveloped the viral nucleocapsids before budding. HBx has transcriptional transactivating potential in the process.

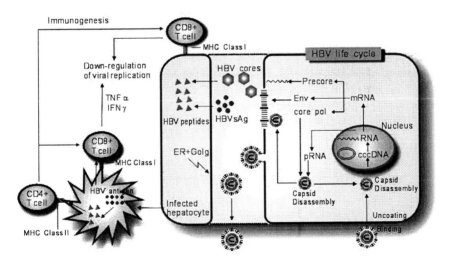

Figure 3.2. The HBV life cycle. Entry of the HBV virion into hepatocyte is a poorly defined process. HBV replicates in the hepatocytes to produce HBsAg particles and virions. The antigens can be recognized by CD8+ or CD4+ T cells, respectively. This recognition reaction can lead to either direct lysis of the infected hepatocyte or the release of interferon and TNF*a*, which can down-regulate viral replication in surrounding hepatocytes without direct cell killing.

The outcome of HBV infection is the result of complicated viral-host interactions [30]. The host's immune attack against HBV is the cause of the liver injury, mediated by a cellular response to small epitopes of HBV proteins, especially HBcAg, presented on the surface of the hepatocyte (figure 3.2).

Human leucocyte antigen (HLA) class I–restricted CD8+ cells recognize HBV peptide fragments derived from intracellular processing and presentation on the hepatocyte surface by class I molecules. This process leads to direct cell killing by the CD8+ cytotoxic T lymphocyte. The evidence suggests that the polymorphic nature of the major-histoco-mpatibility-complex binding sites and differences in the T-cell repertoire among persons leads to highly variable binding affinity for the immunodominant HBV to completion, all infected cells are destroyed, viral replication is aborted, and anti-HBs prevent the reinfection of hepatocytes. If the response is inadequate, the infection continues. However, this is an oversimplification. Sometimes cytotoxic T lymphocytes may directly inhibit viral replication and thus inactivate HBV without killing the infected hepatocyte.

3. Infection

In primary infection, HBsAg becomes detectable in the blood after an incubation period of 2 to 6 months, followed shortly by antibody to HBcAg (anti-HBc). Viremia is well established by the time HBsAg is detected, and titers of virus in acute infection are very high frequently 10^9 to 10^{10} virions per milliliter [31]. In persistent HBV infection, HBsAg remains in the blood and virus production continues, often for life. Reductions in the level of viremia as great as five orders of magnitude may accompany seroconversion to anti-HBe [32]. The table 1 shows typical patterns of serologic and molecular markers in both acute self-limited and chronic HBV infection. We know that at least 70 to 85 percent of people with anti-HBe have detectable viral DNA in the circulation. Although these levels of HBV DNA are relatively low, they are hardly negligible.

Infection with Mutant Viruses

Some HBV variants and specific mutations within the viral genomes might be more frequently associated with the evolution to HCC [33]. The mutation rate of the HBV genome was calculated to 2×10^4 base substitutions per site per year [34]. Naturally occurring mutations have been identified in the structural and non-structural genes as well as regulatory elements of the virus. The best characterized mutants comprise the pre-core (pre-C) stop codon mutation resulting in a loss of

HBeAg, defined clusters of mutations in the core promotor resulting in enhanced viral replication and mutations in the HBcAg and HBsAg altering the antigenicity of the virus. And several mutations in the reverse transcriptase/polymerase genes were identified, conferring resistance to antiviral, and used for the treatment of chronic hepatitis B [35]. The risk of development of LC and HCC is significantly increased in patients with advanced age as well as with basal core-promoter mutant of HBV. In addition, basal core-promoter mutant might contribute to the gender difference of the progression of liver diseases in HBeAg-negative chronic hepatitis B in Taiwan [36]. Combination of pre-S deletion, precore (PC) mutation, and basal core promoter (BCP) mutation rather than single mutation was associated with the development of progressive liver diseases, especially in combination with pre-S deletion. Sequencing analysis showed that the deleted regions were more often in the 3' terminus of pre-S1 and the 5' terminus of pre-S2 [37]. A change in the amino acid sequences at positions 130 and 131 in the HBx protein, such as M130K and V131I, was produced by T-A point mutations at the nucleic acids level, which associated with severe liver damage and HCC in patients from China and Africa [38].

The S-Gene

The clinically most important determinant of HBsAg is the a-determinant (aa 124 to 147), which is now considered to be within a larger antigenic area called the major hydrophilic region (MHR) [39]. The conformation of the a-determinant is a two loop structure which is stabilized by disulphide bridges between Cys-124 and Cys-137 (first loop) and Cys-139 and Cys-147 (second loop).Mutations which abolish the two loop structure of the a-determinant are changes in the hydrophilicity, the electrical charge or the acidity of the loops [40-58]. Mutations nearby the a-determinant [59] might also disturb the secondary structure of the a-determinant.

Deletions within the pre-S1 region can eliminate the promoter of the small-HBsAg. This kind of mutations was found in patients with persistent infections. The large-HBsAg that was encoded by these variant genomes was nonfunctional and the virus maturation was stopped. Deletions which affected the initiation-codon of the pre-S2-mRNA caused an entire loss of the medium-HBsAg. It therefore was speculated that the loss of the highly immunogenic pre-S2-protein is a mechanism to escape the immune system [34, 56, 60, 61].

The Precore-Region

The precore-region plays an important role in viral replication because the pregenomic RNA forms a hairpin structure (NT 1855 to 1858 pair with NT 1896 to 1899) which binds the polymerase. Point mutations of the precore ATG codon have also been observed, which prevent initiation of translation. [62]. The selective disruption of HBeAg expression through mutations affecting the precore region rather than the core gene can be easily understood in terms of the indispensable role of core protein for viral replication. Precore-mutations were found in all forms of infection from asymptomatic carriers [63, 64] to chronic active [65, 66] and fulminant hepatitis [66-72].A G to A mutation at NT 1898 of the precore-region [73] destabilizes the hairpin structure as in genotype A as in genotype D. Therefore it may be disadvantageous for viral replication and consecutively could facilitate integration of HBV-DNA.

The Core-Region

During the asymptomatic period of infection the virus replication is reduced by $CD8^+$ cytotoxic T cells (CTL) whose target is the HBcAg. Mutations inside the CTL-epitopes of the C-gene therefore might create immune escape mutants leading to chronic viral persistence and severe liver disease. A sufficient HBe/HBc specific $CD4^+$ T-cell activity is also considered to be required for an efficient immune response. [74]. Mutations at the codon 130 (Pro to Thr or Ser) might affect the cellular and the humoral immunity because this codon is part of a domain recognized and by B-cells [75] and by T-cells [76].

Core-deletion-mutants mostly were observed in patients with long course infections. The high concentration of polymerase molecules in hepatocytes which are infected with core-deleted HBV might lead to an increased degradation of the polymerase proteins and thereby more antigenic epitopes can be presented to the cytotoxic T-cells.Taken all together the appearance of shortened C-genes in immunocompetent patients could result in a selective disadvantage for the HBV [77].Core-deletion-mutants could be associated with severe liver diseases like cirrhosis and necroinflammation in immunocompromised [78-80] and in immunocompetent patients [77].

The P-Gene

The spacer region was described to be dispensable for the enzyme function and easily tolerates mutations [81, 82]. The catalytic center of the reverse transcriptase was mapped around the aa-sequence YMDD (Tyr –Met – Asp – Asp). This region seems to be the nucleotide recognizing site of the enzyme.

Mutations of the YMDD-sequence were found to be of clinical interest. These mutations within and outsite the YMDD-domain might be selected during lamivudine monotherapy and could contribute to therapy failure [83]. The replication of the Leu-501-variant was at a very low level, which was supposed to be due to a reduced encapsidation of the pregenomic-RNA [84]. Another point mutation which also prevented the encapsidation of the pregenomic-RNA was detected within the RNAseH region of the duck-HBV [85].

The X-Gene

X-deletions which created fusion-proteins between the polymerase and the core-protein (PC-proteins) or between the polymerase and a 3′ truncated HBx (PX-proteins) were found [86]. 3` truncated X-genes were described in acute or chronic hepatitis [87, 88] and in cells from hepatocellular carcinomas. HBx mutants with a COOH-terminal deletion enhanced transforming ability of ras and myc. Natural HBx mutants might be selected in tumor tissues and play a role in hepatocarcinogenesis by modifying the biological functions of HBx. X-mutants might cause important problems in blood donors. They are suspected to lead to a transmissible HBV infection which cannot be detected by conventional test systems because the classical serological markers HBsAg and HBeAg can be missing.Furthermore many X-deletions were described to affect the precore-start-codon thus leading to a HBeAg-negative serotype [89,90]. On the other hand the X-deletion-mutants may interfere with the replication and the packaging of the wild type virus and thereby reduce the serum level of the wild type HBV [89].From the described course of infection it might be concluded that anti-HBs is not protective against X-deletion-mutants. This might explain that HBV can chronically persist after the seroconversion to antiHBs-positive [90].

4. Coinfection of HBV and HDV, HCV or HIV

Hepatitis D

Hepatitis D virus (HDV) [91,92] is a defective, RNA-containing passenger virus requiring the helper functions provided by HBV, including nucleocapsid assembly and provision of an HBsAg derived envelope.HDV infection occurs either as a simultaneous coinfection with HBV or as a superinfection in an HBV carrier, typically an injection-drug user. HDV infection is an important consideration when the condition of a patient with chronic HBV infection worsens or when a test for HBeAg is negative but active liver disease persists.[93,94] Patients with HBV-HDV coinfection may have more severe acute disease and a higher risk of fulminant hepatitis (2%-20%) compared with those infected with HBV alone.In long-term studies of chronic HBV carriers with HDV superinfection, 70%-80% have developed evidence of chronic liver diseases with cirrhosis compared with 15%-30% of patients with chronic HBV infection alone.

Hepatitis C

As HBV and hepatitis C virus (HCV) share similar transmission routes, coinfection with the two viruses is not a rare event in intravenous drug users and in countries with a high prevalence of HBV [95,96]. Many injection-drug users have detectable antibody to HBcAg and HCV, indicating exposure to both parenteral hepatotropic viruses. Although HBV is cleared in most adults, approximately 90 percent have active hepatitis C, and a smaller fraction (approximately 5 percent) have dual infections, with very active liver disease. These coinfections accelerate the course of chronic liver disease and facilitate progression to cirrhosis and hepatocellular carcinoma [97-101]. Some data suggest a more than additive but less than multiplicative effect of HBV and HCV coinfection on the relative risk for HCC. The viruses may act through common as well as different pathways in the carcinogenic process [102]. Clinical data obtained from chronic HBV carriers superinfected with HCV suggest that HCV may inhibit HBV replication. Some studies have shown that HCV core and NS2 proteins inhibit HBV replication and gene expression in vitro [103-105].

Human Immunodeficiency Virus

Because the diseases are spread in similar ways—notably through shared use of needles to inject drugs and sexual activity—many people are coinfected with, HIV and HBV. Most studies show that HIV infection leads to more aggressive hepatitis B and a higher risk of liver damage. The relationship between coinfection and risk was strongest in the setting of low CD4+ cell count and with treatment in the post-antiretroviral therapy treatment era. Viral clearance in the form of conversion to HBV surface antigen-negative (HBsAg-) status, is a rare event in coinfected patients.

Studies of how HBV affect HIV disease are less clear. Coinfection can complicate treatment. People with liver damage due to chronic hepatitis are more likely to experience hepatotoxicity (liver toxicity) related to anti-HIV drugs. In addition, drugs used to treat HIV and hepatitis can interact and side effects may be exacerbated. HBV infection was not treated in HIV-positive persons because of their limited life expectancy; improvements in survival and new agents that are effective against one or both of the viruses have made treatment possible.[106,107] Therapeutic agents active against both viruses should be utilized at the correct dose to limit the development of resistance [108,109].

II. Pathogenesis of Hepatocellular Carcinoma

HBV infection is a risk factor for hepatocellular carcinoma, which arises almost exclusively in patients with cirrhosis. As with other forms of liver cancer, tumors associated with hepatitis B result from chronic inflammation and repeated cellular regeneration, typically occurring only after 25 to 30 years of infection. [110,111]

HCC incidence is three to four times higher in males than in females, suggesting a tumorigenic effect of androgens [112,113]. A recent study suggested positive HBsAg increased one's risk of developing HCC by 10 folds, and with positive HBeAg, HCC is significantly increased by 60 folds. Moreover, a detectable HBV DNA level yields a 4 fold increase risk of HCC [114]. The additional use of alcohol, consumption of aflatoxin in diet and coinfection with HCV or HDV are independent factors for HCC in HBV infected patients (table 1).

Table 1. Independent Risk Factors
for the Development of HCC in HBV Infection

Types	Risk Factors
Host	Male
	Older age(>45 years old)
	First degree relatives with HCC
Clinical	HBeAg positive
	Detectable HBV DNA
	Cirrhosis
	Persistent HBV infection
	(HBsAg positive)
Viral and environmental	Coinfection with HCV or HDV
	Alcohol intake
	Aflatoxin in Diet

The mechanisms responsible for malignant transformation in chronic HBV infection are not well defined, and both viral and host factors have been implicated in the process [115]. Various viral factors associated with hepatocellular carcinoma development include HBV genotype, basal core promoter mutations, and high viral load.

Polymorphisms at the androgen receptor-regulating genes and cytokine genes are possible host factors associated with HCC [116]. On the one hand, all cases of HCC occur after many years of chronic hepatitis which could, theoretically, provide the mitogenic [117] and mutagenic environment to precipitate random genetic and chromosomal damage, and lead to the development of HCC [118,119]. Some results have shown that high percentages of hepatocytes showing nucleolar hypertrophy significantly predict HCC development in patients with HBV infection [120]. Centrosome abnormalities, such as excess number or variable shape and size, have been found in human cancer of multiple origins [121]. HBx induced centrosome hyperamplification and mitotic aberration by activation of the Ras-MEK-MAPK, which may contribute to genomic instability during hepatocarcinogenesis [122]. On the other hand, most tumors contain clonally integrated HBV DNA and microdeletions in the flanking cellular DNA that could, theoretically, deregulate cellular growth control mechanisms. Integration of HBV DNA occurred frequently in HCC and LC cases with chronic HBV infection, whereas HBx integration occurred more often in HCC than in LC cases [123]. The integrated viral DNA might therefore act as a mutagenic agent, followed by causing secondary chromosomal rearrangement, such as duplications, translocations, deletions, and increasing genomic instability [124,125]. Interestingly HBV-DNA from liver tissues especially from hepatocellular carcinoma cells was found to possess more mutants than HBVDNA from the serum [41, 73, 126]. Furthermore, The HBV DNA integration and its gene mutation on precore region and p53 gene mutation probably play synergic roles in the development of HCC [127].

Hepatitis B Virus X (HBx) Protein and Pathogenensis of HCC

A clinical study demonstrated that 40.0% of sera and 85% of liver tissues from HCC patients tested positive for HBxAg. In addition, 70.0% of sera from HCC patients tested positive for anti-HBx antibody [128]. In our study we found that HBxAg was highly expressed in the cytoplasm of cells found in liver tumor tissues (76.5%) and cirrhosis tissues (100%) [129]. Expression of anti-HBx antibody in sera correlated well with markers of HBV replication, such as HBsAg and HBcAg proteins [130]. Taken together, these data suggest that monitoring of HBx anti-HBx antibody in serum could be useful for early diagnosis and prognosis in patients with chronic HBV infection, LC, and HCC. [131,132]

HBx protein is multifunctional viral protein. HCC cells containing HBx protein have enhanced invasive potential conditionally.[133] Since HBx interacts with and stimulates many kinases, such as PKC, Jak1, IKK, PI-3-K, NF-κB, SAPK and Akt/PKB, it has been speculated that HBx might act as an adaptor or kinase activator, enhancing the phosphorylation of HBx-associated proteins. A possible interaction of HBx with the mitochondrion is also intriguing. Biologically elucidating the significant activity of HBx may give further insight into the role of HBx and ultimately lead to new therapeutic strategies for managing HBV-related HCC patients as well as contribute to the clinical therapy of HCC.

HBx and Regulation of Apoptosis

Apoptosis is necessary for the elimination of redundant, damaged and virally infected cells. HBx affects the regulation of apoptosis through its action on caspases, mitochondria and survivin[134,135]. Apoptosis induced by ectopic expression of HBx is associated with mitochondrial membrane alterations and caspase 3 activation [134]. HBx has been demonstrated to efficiently block caspase 3 (CPP32) activity and apoptosis in both rat fibroblasts and hepatoma cells [135] HBx perturbs intracellular Ca^{2+} homeostasis by acting on caspase-3-dependent extrusion mechanisms. This effect plays an important role in the control of HBx-related apoptosis [136]. And some findings suggest that HBx sensitizes primary mouse hepatocytes to ethanol- and TNF-alpha-induced apoptosis by a caspase-3-dependent mechanism, which may partly explain the synergistic effects of alcohol consumption and hepatitis B virus infection on liver injury. [137]

HBx has been demonstrated to localize to the mitochondria. *In vivo* studies also suggest it plays a role in apoptosis, possibly by interacting with Bcl-2 during hepatic apoptosis. It is also been suggested that in hepatitis B virus-infected cells, the location of HBx in mitochondria can cause the loss of mitochondrial membrane potential, subsequently inducing mitochondria-dependent cell death.

Survivin is a protein which inhibits apoptosis and is overexpressed in most human cancers [138]. Studies in our laboratory suggest that HBx can up-regulate the expression of survivin in hepatic carcinoma cells, inhibiting apoptosis of hepatic carcinoma cells induced by adriamycin [139]. Survivin–hepatitis B X-interacting protein (HBXIP) complexes bind pro-caspase-9 preventing its action on Apaf-1 and consequently suppressing apoptosis initiated via the mitochondria/cytochrome c pathway. Viral HBx also been shown to interact with the survivin–HBXIP complex, suppressing caspase activation in a survivin-dependent manner [140]. Our study suggests that survivin may be a co-factor of HBx in transformation of hepatocytes induced by HBx. It is likely that these proteins act in concert to induce aberrant mitosis and genomic instability of host hepatic cells.

Effects of HBx on Signal Pathways

Intracellular localization studies have demonstrated that HBx is localized to both the cytoplasm and the nucleus [141,142]. It can influence transcriptional activators and activate many cellular and viral transcriptional elements [143-148]. For example, HBx upregulates the transcriptional activity of proto-oncogenes (c-Myc, N-myc and c-jun) and transcription factors such as activating protein-1 (AP-1), NF-κB, and the ATF/cAMP response element-binding protein (CREB)[149-151,156-158]. Some gene networks analysis showed that activation of AP-1 transcription factors in a newly identified HCC subtype might play a key role in tumor development [152]. Furthermore, some results suggest that the interaction between HBx and Jun activation domain-binding protein 1 (Jab1) enhances HBx-mediated AP-1 activation.[153] HBx has also been found to be associated with a great number of genes, such as tumor necrosis factor (TNF), transforming growth factor β1 (TGF-β1), epidermal growth factor (EGF) receptor, interleukin 8 (IL-8), and p53, among others [154]. It has also been demonstrated that HBx can interact with nucleotide excision DNA repair pathway [155]. Recent studies suggest that HBx expression in HepG2 cells regulated the expression of 39 genes [134], including cell cycle regulate genes, oncogenes, and apoptosis effectors.

HBx has been shown to upregulate the Ras-Raf-mitogen-activated protein kinase (MAPK) signal cascade [156-160]. HBx-mediated RAS-RAF-MAPK pathway activation is also associated with accelerating entry of cells into S phase [161], detrimentally affecting the cell cycle. Importantly, data suggest that CREB is the downstream target of the RAS-RAF-MAPK pathway, as studies have demonstrated that CREB phosphorylation, *in vivo,* is mediated by HBx-dependent activation of the RAS-RAF-MAPK pathway. In other cell lines, HBx-dependent activation of p38 MAPK inactivates Cdc25C by phosphorylation of Ser216, and then initiates activation of the G_2/M checkpoint, which may delay cell growth. Interestingly, it has been also shown that HBx upregulates Src kinase that is subsequently tyrosine phosphorylated to activate Ras. Src tyrosine kinase activation not only changes the expression of Ras *in vivo*, but can also influence HBV replication by stimulating the activity of viral polymerase [162,163].

Phosphatidylinositol 3-kinase (PI-3-K) and its downstream target, protein kinase B (PKB)/Akt, are induced by many factors, such as TGF-β, to inhibit apoptosis. HBx downregulates TGF-β-induced apoptosis in hepatocytes by stimulating PI-3-K activity [164]. The activation of PI-3-K signaling pathway is attributed, at least in part, to the anti-apoptotic mechanism of HBx [165]. It has also been demonstrated that HBx activates other signaling pathways, such as the Src kinase-Ras-GTP complex [166] and the Jak1-signal transducer and activator of transcription (STAT) that activate the PI-3-K-Akt/PKB pathway indirectly. Taken together, these data indicate that the hepatitis B virus inhibits apoptotic death through an HBx-PI-3-K-Akt-Bad-dependant pathway.

Some results suggest that HBx is an inducer of the Jak-STAT signaling pathway [167]. Additional studies reveal that some HBx mutants that differ from their association from of the wild-type HBx lose the ability to activate STAT-3 and NF-κB. In HepG2 cells transfected with the wild-type HBx expression vector, the level of tyrosine phosphorylation of STAT-3 was activated by HBx [168]. Stimulation of growth factors, during partial hepatectomy, results in the activation of JAK/STAT signaling, in the liver, and has been associated with increased hepatocyte proliferation [169,170]. Because of its ability to induce Src PTK, HBx protein may have many effects on transforming cellular processes.

It has been reported that HBx is an activator of transcription factor NF-κB, which was one of the first HBx-responsive motifs to be identified [150,151]. Some people find that HBx up-regulates lymphotoxin alpha (LTalpha) expression at the transcriptional level through an NF-kappaB-dependent mechanism and, therefore, the up-regulated LTalpha may be secreted and involved in the HBx-induced NF-κB activation.[171] NF-κB stimulated by HBx promotes the survival of liver cells against Fas-mediated apoptosis[172]. HBx can directly bind with IκB subunit of the NF-κB complex, causing HBx to enter the nucleus [170]. The ability of NF-κB to mediate apoptosis was inhibited HBx-expressing cells, a fact which may play a central role in programmed cell death [173,174]. An overwhelming of evidence indicates that the Wnt signaling pathway play a crucial role during the development of many organs. Several studies suggest that enhanced expression of NF-κB-associated Wnt-1 protein might be a mechanism of hepatocarcinogenesis common to HBV- and HCV-infected patients. NF-κB signaling pathway and Wnt-1 protein could be potential targets for designing highly effective therapeutic agents in treating HCC and for chemoprevention of hepatocarcinogenesis. [175,176]

Effect of HBx on Cell Cycle

Several studies have shown that HBx can affect cell cycle checkpoints [177]. Many genes involved in cell cycle regulation (cyclins, kinases, negative regulators, Wnt-β-catenin) and the transcription profile are altered in most HCC patients [178]. HBx is able to upregulate the activation rate and level of the cyclin-dependent kinase (CDK) 2 and CDC2, as well as enhance their active association with cyclin E and cyclin A or cyclin B, respectively. HBx protein can block G1/S transition of the hepatocyte cell-cycle progression and causes both a failure of liver functionality and cell death in the regenerating liver of the HBx transgenic mice. [179] The effect of HBx on the G_1–S checkpoint control depends on the status of p53. Transcription of $p21^{wafl/cip1}$ has been demonstrated to be activated by HBx, in the presence of functional p53 and in a dose-dependent manner. However, the same transcription was depressed by HBx when p53 was absent or present at a low level. Furthermore, HBx has been shown to activate the cyclin A promoter, induce cyclin A-cyclin-dependent kinase 2 complexes and promote cycling of growth-arrested cells into G_1, a reaction which also depends the Src tyrosine kinases-activating pathway. HBx stimulation of Src kinases and cyclin gene expression was found to force growth-arrested cells to transit through G_1 but to stall at the junction with S phase [180]. Some studys show that HBx up-regulates cyclin D1 and this process is mediated by the NF-κB2(p52)/BCL-3 complex. This HBx-mediated-cyclin D1 up-regulation might play an important role in the HBx-mediated HCC development and progression. [181]

HBx and hTERT

Telomere length becomes stabilized in most tumor cells, highly proliferating cells and human somatic cells, by the activation of telomerase. The most crucial catalytic protein subunit of telomerase ribonuclear protein is human telomerase reverse transcriptase (hTERT), whose expression parallels telomerase activity [182]. hTERT expression is regulated mainly at the transcriptional level and the core promoter of hTERT contains many binding sites for transcription factors. [183]. A study has shown that HBV DNA integration is located upstream to the hTERT promoter and that the HBV enhancer can cis-activate the transcriptional expression of hTERT gene in hepatocarcinoma cell lines [184]. Experiments in our laboratory have found that both HBxAg and telomerase were highly expressed in hepatoma tissues and liver cirrhosis tissues. Additionally, HBx gene can upregulate the expression and activity of hTERT, suggesting that HBx expression may play a role in hepatocellular carcinogenesis by interfering with telomerase activity during hepatocyte proliferation [185]. These findings suggest a new mechanism of HBV in liver carcinogenesis.

HBx and Damaged DNA-Binding Complex

DNA damage may be an initiating factor in hepatocarcinogenesis and that HBx may act as the promoting factor by inhibiting DNA repair. In hepatitis B virus-infected hepatocytes, a chronic infection may present the opportunity for such a DNA-damaging event to occur, and accumulated errors caused by the inhibition of DNA repair by HBx may result in oncogenesis.[186] Damaged DNA binding protein (DDB) has been demonstrated to contribute to DNA repair. DDB2 transports DDB1 from the cytoplasm to the nucleus [187,188]. The DDB1 subunit of UV-DDB is a cellular target for HBx. Hepatitis B virus X protein can stimulate viral genome replication via a DDB1-dependent pathway distinct from that leading to cell death.[189] HBx may simultaneously bind to both subunits of DDB to form a X-DDB1-DDB2 complex, that is, DDB1 prominently increases HBx stability while DDB2 relieves this effect. It has also been shown that physical interactions occurring within the X-DDB1-DDB2 complex mediate these effects through the modulation of proteasome-dependent degradation of HBx [190]. DDB2 is expressed only during late-G_1 phase, consequently, the DDB2-mediated accumulation of HBx during late-G_1 phase may be crucial for viral replication, from which the host cell then produces the replication proteins and enzymes during that phase of the cell cycle [191]. The effect of HBx on signal pathways was summarized in figure 4.

HBx Binding Proteins

It has been demonstrated that activating transcription factor 2 (ATF2) inhibits basal transcription of the X promoter and the transactivation activity of HBx through activating protein-1 (AP-1). Although the X promoter was shown to be repressed by ATF2, the small X promoter had an ATF2 binding site and was stimulated by ATF2 [192]. It was also reported that HBx specifically interacts with TATA-binding protein (TBP) *in vitro*. The binding interaction between HBx and p53 has been previously identified and it was demonstrated that the C-terminal region of HBx is required for maintaining the p53 in the cytoplasm and suppressing p53-mediated apoptosiss [193]. Some results demonstrate that HBx can destroy the ability of p53 to regulate α-fetoprotein (AFP) in a tissue-specific manner [194], but later some studies have found that serum AFP levels in HCC patients are not influenced by virus B or C hepatitis pattern and AFP dosage should not be used for HCC diagnosis in non-cirrhotic patients [195].

HBx directly interacts with the bZip transactivator CREB and the basic region/leucine zipper (bZip) repressors ICER IIg and ATF3, increasing their ability to bind to DNA *in vitro* as well as their transcriptional efficacy *in vivo* [196]. It has also been found that HBx interacts with many other members of the bZip group of dimerizing leucine zipper transcriptional factors, gadd153/Chop10 and NF-IL6, which may activate or repress gene expression in the liver [196]. Qadri I et al. [197] demonstrated that HBx binds with TFIIH complexes both *in vitro* and *in vivo*. Furthermore, HBx and RNA polymerase II subunit 5 (RPB5) interact with other general transcription factors. HBx and RPB5 both specifically bind to transcription factor TFIIB. Delineation of the binding regions of these three proteins revealed that HBx, RPB5 and TFIIB each have two binding regions for the other two proteins. The transactivation of HBx requires the interaction of both RPB5 and TFIIB [198].

The direct binding between HBx and human voltage-dependent anion channel 3 (HVDAC3) has also been demonstrated. A HVDAC3 and HBx complex was colocalized to mitochondria and the mitochondrial association of HBx contributes to the alteration of the mitochondrial trans-membrane potential [199]. The region necessary for HBx's mitochondrial localization was located to amino acids 68–117, which is essential for cell death but inactive for transactivation function [200].

HBx can also interact with the proteasome complex. It has been previously shown that a proteasome subunit, PSMA7 is a putative cellular target of HBx [201,202]. It is also reported that another HBx-interacting subunit similar to the proteasome subunit PSMC1, an ATPase-like member of the 19 S regulatory factor [203-205], has been identified interacting with HBx. The interacting domains of PSMA7, PSMC1 and HBx have been mapped and the specificity of these interactions was also further evaluated using a modified yeast two-hybrid dissociator system [206].

Heat shock protein 60 (Hsp60) and heat shock protein 70 (Hsp70) have also been identified as a cellular target of HBx. Hsp60 and HBx provide a mechanism for the control of the proapoptotic function of HBx. [207] A research suggests that HBx can directly bind to Hsp70, demonstrating that HBx can form a complex with Hsp60 and Hsp70. Further research is needed to fully elucidate the implications of a HBx, Hsp60 and Hsp70 complex in the molecular mechanism of action of viral infections. [208] Studies shown that hTid-1 and Hdj1, the human Hsp40/DnaJ chaperone proteins, bind the HBV core protein and inhibit viral replication in cell culture system. Furthermore several evidences suggest that HBX is the major target of Hdj1 in the inhibition of HBV replication. These results might provide a molecular basis for the antiviral effect of cellular chaperones. [209,210]

The research of the role of HBx *in vivo* in the viral life cycle should go some ways to understanding the mechanism of HCC that is associated with chronic HBV infection [129,131,139,211]. A paracrine effect of viral proteins on cell transformation and angiogenesis has been hypothesized for only a few human viruses implicated in carcinogenesis. Some findings demonstrate that HBx may in fact act by combining intracellular and paracrine effects, and inhibiting the proliferation of both infected and uninfected liver cells in the context of liver regeneration. This dual property would have a selective effect, promoting the expansion of cells resistant to the inhibitory effect of HBx [212].

Gelatinase, matrix metalloproteinase (MMP) -2 and 9, plays an important role in the pathogenesis of LC and HCC [213,214]. Some results clearly suggest that the HBx contributed to the transcriptional regulation of MMP-9 through the ERKs and PI-3K-AKT/PKB pathways, and increased an invasive potential of cells [215]. Some results indicate that the AFP level and ratio of MMP-9/MMP-2 are highly correlated to chronic HBV-induced hepatitis. Because the serum MMP activities were significantly varied between each stage of AFP production in liver disease, an individual profile of these parameters might serve as an easy accessing serum marker to monitor the progression of liver disease [216]. Trans-activation proficient HBx up-regulated the transcription, translation and secretion of matrix metalloproteinase-3 (MMP-3), manifest as a cell migratory phenotype. This HBx effect was abrogated in the presence of a MMP-3 specific peptide inhibitor. So

HBx exerts selective transcriptional control in hepatoma cells and induces cellular migration through the activation of MMP-3. [217]

The progression of chronic hepatitis B is related to fibrosis and to the emergence of intrahepatic anomalous vascular structures. HBx may play a significant role in both processes. HBx could account for the induction of Ang2 observed in chronic hepatitis B, especially the 50-kd form, contributing to pathological angiogenesis and hepatocellular carcinoma progression. [189] Recent study suggests that HBx plays a role during hepatocellular carcinogenesis by favoring cell detachment from the surrounding cells and migration outside of the primary tumor site. [218]

Estrogen, which exerts its biological function through estrogen receptor (ER), can inhibit HBV replication. ERDelta5, an ERalpha variant lacking exon 5, was found to be preferentially expressed in patients with HCC compared with patients with normal livers. Data suggest that HBx and ERDelta5 may play a negative role in ERalpha signaling and that ERalpha agonists may be developed for HCC therapy. [219]

Macrophage migration inhibitory factor (MIF) is implicated in the regulation of inflammation, cell growth, and even tumor formation. Both HBx and MIF cause HepG2 cell G_0/G_1 phase arrest, proliferation inhibition, and apoptosis. However, MIF can counteract the apoptotic effect of HBx. These results may provide evidence to explain the link between HBV infection and hepatocellular carcinoma. [220]

The up-regulation of proteasome subunits and lysosomal proteases in hepatocellular carcinomas of the HBx gene knockin transgenic mice.All these results suggested that the strengthened ubiquitin-proteasome and lysosomal pathway might contribute to the development of HBx-related HCC. [221]

III. Systems to Study the Biological Properties of HBV

In Vitro Model Systems

A major obstacle to the research on the development of drug and gene-based therapies for HBV infections has been the lack of an efficient cell culture system or a readily available small-animal model, permissive for viral infection and replication. Fortunately, numerous strategies have been employed, including

HBV transfected cell lines, such as 2.2.15 cells. [222,223] Ladner *et al.* have developed a cell line, designated HepAD38, in which the replication of HBV can be regulated with tetracycline [224,225]. Another cell system, HepAD79, has also been developed to determine the relative susceptibility of viruses with mutations in the YMDD motif in cell culture [224]. Additionally, HBV-infected primary human hepatocyte cultures, as well as primary duck hepatocyte (PDH) cultures infected with duck hepatitis B virus (DHBV) have been used for the evaluation of antiviral agents. [226] A partial list of existing cell culture models appears in table 2.

Table 2. Models to Study HBV Infection

Cell culture models
* Infection of primary hepatocytes
* Stable transfection of hepatocyte cell lines
* Surrogate models
Hepadna viruses: Woodchuck hapatocytes for WHV
Duck hapatocytes for DHV
In vivo models
* Chimpanzee(Pan troglodytes)
* Tupaia belengeri sinensis
* Transgenic mice
* Immunodeficient mice or tolerized rates transplanted with
Human hepatocytes
* Surrogate models
Woodchuck for WHV; Pekin duck for DBV;tamarins for GB
Virus A and B(GBV-A,B);ground squirrel for GSHV

In Vivo Models

The availability of animal models for the study of hepatitis B virus (HBV) infection has assisted the discovery of the molecular mechanism of genome replication, viral persistence, and pathogenesis.

Chimpanzees

Chimpanzees have been shown to be exquisitely susceptible to human hepatitis viruses, without themselves developing clinical illness, thus providing an important model for studies on these agents. Before embarking on development of vaccines and therapies, virologists must characterize the biological properties of target viruses. Examples of such studies carried out in chimpanzees follow.

These studies were an essential prerequisite for subsequent vaccine development and evaluation in the chimpanzee model. Because no in vitro assay was available for detection of infectious HBV, use of the chimpanzee was the only way to ensure that lapses of Good Manufacturing Practice did not result in batches of plasma-derived HBV vaccine containing live HBV.

Researchers demonstrated that ~3–6% of the wild-caught chimpanzees were positive for HBsAg, and ~50% of the older animals were positive for the antibody to HBsAg, a marker for resolved HBV infection. [227] The thinking was that these HBV infections resulted from the practice of injecting human serum in wild-caught animals to improve their survival during transit and confinement; however, various groups have recently demonstrated the presence of a unique chimpanzee HBV strain that was verified by sequencing of the entire genome. [228-230] Chimpanzees inoculated with HBsAg+ chimpanzee plasma developed characteristic hepatitis, HBs antigenemia, and eventual anti-HBs seroconversion.

Chimpanzees have contributed immensely in the development of HBV vaccines, evaluation of the safety of blood products, and the discovery of HCV. However, their limited availability, expense, endangered status, and the lack of chronic liver disease precludes the study of pathogenesis of cirrhosis and HCC. It is also not practical to use chimpanzees for the preclinical evaluation of novel drugs and therapies of viral hepatitis.

The Tupaia

Tree shrews (*Tupaia belangeri sinensis*) are nonrodent small animals that are phylogenetically close to primates. They adapt easily to a laboratory environment. Apart from the chimpanzee, the tree shrews are the only other animals that HBV can infect. [231,232] The early steps of HBV infection in tupaia hepatocytes are very similar to those in human hepatocytes, with both pre-S1 and S antigens being necessary for infection [233]. However, the efficiency of HBV infection is low, and it has been reported that human serum interferes with HBV binding to the tupaia hepatocytes [234]. Researchers have examined in tupaias the hepatocarcinogenic effects of HBV infection alone and in combination with dietary aflatoxins [235,236]. The incidence of HCC was significantly higher in the animals that were both infected with HBV and exposed to aflatoxin (52.94%) than in those solely infected with HBV (11.11%) or exposed to aflatoxin B1 (12.50%)[236]. In contrast to control animals, precancerous lesions, including liver cell dysplasia and enzyme-altered hyperplastic hepatocyte foci, were evident before the occurrence of HCC, and the frequency of their appearance correlated well with the incidence of HCC [236].

Rodent Models

Experimental models to study effects of drugs on HBV replication were described using nude mice [237,238]. These mice were inoculated with HBV-transfected hepatoma cell lines. The resulting models are suitable to study tumour formation rather than chronic HBV infection. Feitelson and colleagues have recently reported a transgenic SCID mouse model in which the mice reliably developed chronic liver disease. Such HBV transgenic SCID mice have continuous evidence of gene expression and virus replication in both serum and liver throughout their life-spans. This system offers a reproducible model of chronic liver disease, and could be useful in evaluating antiviral agents for HBV in a small animal model.

Tolerized Rats

Tolerant rats with chimeric human livers could be infected with HBV.Normal rats were tolerized to human hepatocytes by exposure to human hepatocytes at day 17 of gestation. Tolerant animals with transplanted human hepatocytes were susceptible to HBV infection.

Surrogate Animal Models: Woodchuck, Duck, Ground Squirrel

Researchers have used naturally occurring HBV-like viruses, such as the ground squirrel hepatitis virus (GSHV) that infects ground squirrels, [239] the duck hepatitis B virus (DHV) that infects Pekin ducks, [240] and the woodchuck hepatitis virus (WHV) that infects woodchucks, [241] to investigate viral DNA integration and to assess antiviral therapies [242]. WHV induces HCC in its host. [241] The mechanism of WHV- and HBV-induced HCC seems to consist of many steps. HCC in chronically infected woodchucks occurs more frequently than in ground squirrels chronically infected with GSHV. [243] The woodchuck model has contributed importantly to the understanding of viral replication, chronic infection, and hepatic carcinogenicity of hepadnaviruses. However, the lack of inbred strains and of immunological reagents to study lymphocyte subsets in woodchucks remains a formidable obstacle to investigation of the immunological pathogenesis of viral hepatitis. Immunotherapeutic agents against WHV will not be effective against HBV, and vaccines against HBV can never be tested in woodchucks. Furthermore, these animals do not develop cirrhosis. Therefore, there are limitations to the types of experiments that could be devised to investigate the mechanisms of pathogenesis of viral hepatitis.

Although no single cell culture system or animal model is ideal for studying all features of HBV hepatitis, researchers are developing imaginative and novel animal models that are designed to investigate specific aspects of pathobiology, prevention, and therapy of HBV.

References

[1]   Chisari FV. (2000).Viruses, immunity, and cancer: lessons from hepatitis B. *Am. J. Pathol*, 156(4):1117-1132.

[2]   Villeneuve JP. (2005).The natural history of chronic hepatitis B virus infection. *J. Clin. Virol*, 34 (Suppl 1):S139-142.

[3]   Chu CM. (2000).Natural history of chronic hepatitis B virus infection in adults with emphasis on the occurrence of cirrhosis and hepatocellular carcinoma. *J. Gastroenterol. Hepatol*, 15(Supp l): E25-30.

[4]   Carman WF, Jacyna MR, Hadziyannis S et al.(1989) Mutation preventing formation of hepatitis B e antigen in patients with chronic hepatitis B infection. *Lancet*, 2(8663):588–591.

[5]   Marcellin P, Castelnau C, Martinot-Peignoux M, et al. (2005).Natural history of hepatitis B. *Minerva Gastroenterol Dietol*, 51(1):63-75.

[6]   Yim HJ, Lok AS.(2006).Natural history of chronic hepatitis B virus infection: what we knew in 1981 and what we know in 2005. *Hepatology*, 43(2Suppl1):S173-181.

[7]   de Jongh FE, Janssen HL, de Man RA, et al.(1992).Survival and prognostic indicators in hepatitis B surface antigen-positive cirrhosis of liver. *Gastroenterology*, 103(5):1630-1635.

[8]   de Jongh FE, Giustina G, Schalm SW, et al. (1995). Occurrence of hepatocellular carcinoma and decompensation in western European patients with cirrhosis type B. *Hepatology*, 21(1):77-82.

[9]   Kao JH, Chen PJ, Lai MY, et al.(2000).Hepatitis B genotypes correlate with clinical outcomes in patients with chronic hepatitis B. *Gastroenterology*, 118(3):554-559.

[10]   Chu CM, Liaw YF. (2006). Hepatitis B virus-related cirrhosis: natural history and treatment. *Semin. Liver Dis* , 26(2): 142-52.

[11]   Eckert DM, Kim PS. (2001).Mechanism of viral membrane fusion and its inhibition. *Annu. Rev. Biochem*, 70:777-810.

[12]   Lobigs M,Garoff H.(1990). Fusion function of Semliki Forest virus spike is activated by proteolytic cleavage of the envelope glycoprotein precursor P62. *J. Virol*, 64(3): 1233-1240.

[13]   Stibbe W, Gerlich WH. (1983).Structural relationships between minor and major proteins of hepatitis B surface antigen. *J. Virol*, 46(2): 626-628.

[14]   Heermann KH, Goldmann U, Schwartz W, Seyffarth T, Baumgarten H, Gerlich WH.(1984).Large surface proteins of hepatitis B virus containing the pre-S sequence. *J. Virol*, 52(2): 396- 402.

[15]   Neurath AR, Seto B, Strick N.(1989).Antibodies to synthetic peptides from the PreS I region of the hepatitis B virus (HBV) envelope (env) protein are virus neutralizing and protective. *Vaccine*, 7(3): 234-236.

[16]   Neurath AR, Kent SB, Strick N, Parker K.(1986).Identification and chemical synthesis of a host cell receptor binding site on hepatitis B virus. *Cell*, 46(3): 429-436.

[17]   Bruss V, Ganem D.(1991).The role of envelope proteins in hepatitis B virus assembly. *Proc. Natl. Acad. Sci. USA*, 88(3):1059-1063.

[18]   Paran N, Geiger B, and Shaul Y. (2001). HBV infection of cell culture: evidence for multivalent and cooperative attachment. *EMBO J*,20(16):4443-4453.

[19]   Pontisso P, Petit MA, Bankowski MJ, and Peeples ME. (1989). Human
        liver plasma membranes contain receptors for the hepatitis B virus pre-S1
        region and, via polymerized human serum albumin, for the pre-S2 region.
        J. Virol,63(5): 1981-1988.
[20]   de Bruin W, Leenders W, Kos T, Hertogs K, Depla E, Yap SH.(1994).
        Hepatitis delta virus attaches to human hepatocytes via human liver
        endonexin II, a specific HBsAg binding protein. *J. Viral. Hepat*, 1(1): 33-
        38.
[21]   Treichel U, Meyer Z, Buschenfelde KH, Dienes HP, Gerken
        G.(1997).Receptor-mediated entry of hepatitis B virus particles into liver
        cells. *Arch. Virol*, 142(3): 493-498.
[22]   Peeples ME, Komai K, Radek R, Bankowski MJ.(1987).A cultured cell
        receptor for the small S protein of hepatitis B virus. *Virology*,160(1): 135-
        142.
[23]   Gerlich WH, Lu X, Heermann KH.(1993).Studies on the attachment and
        penetration of hepatitis B virus. *J. Hepatol*, 17 (Suppl. 3):S10-S14.
[24]   Hughson FM. (1995).Structural characterization of viral fusion proteins.
        Curr. Biology, 5(3): 265-274.
[25]   Rose OD, Roy S. (1980).Hydrophobic basis of packing in globular
        proteins. *Proc. Natl. Acad. Sci. USA*, 77(8): 4643-4647.
[26]   Dimitrov AS, Xiao X, Dimitrov DS, Blumenthal R. (2001).Early
        intermediates in HIV-1 envelope glycoproteinmediated fusion triggered
        by CD4 and co-receptor complexes. *Journal of Biological Chemistry*,
        276(32): 30335-30341.
[27]   Formanowski F, Wharton SA, Calder LJ, Hofbauer C, Meier-Ewert H.
        (1990).Fusion characteristics of influenza C viruses. *J. Gen. Virol*,
        71(Pt5): 1181-1188.
[28]   Breiner KM, Schaller H. (2000).Cellular receptor traffic is essential for
        productive duck hepatitis B virus infection. *J. Virol*, 74(5): 2203-2209.
[29]   Guo JT, Pugh JC. (1997).Monoclonal antibodies to a 55-kilodalton
        protein present in duck liver inhibit infection of primary duck hepatocytes
        with duck hepatitis B virus. *J. Virol*, 71(6): 4829-4831.
[30]   Rapicetta M, Ferrari C, Levrero M.(2002).Viral determinants and host
        immune responses in the pathogenesis of HBV infection. *J. Med. Virol*,
        67(3), 454-457.
[31]   Ribeiro RM, Lo A, Perelson AS.(2002).Dynamics of hepatitis B virus
        infection. *Microbes Infect*, 4(8): 829-835.

[32]   Tedder RS, Ijaz S, Gilbert N, et al.(2002).Evidence for a dynamic host-
parasite relationship in e-negative hepatitis B carriers. *J. Med. Virol*,
68(4): 505-512.

[33]   Pujol FH, Devesa M. (2005). Genotypic variability of hepatitis viruses
associated with chronic infection and the development of hepatocellular
carcinoma. *J. Clin. Gastroenterol*, 39(7):611-618.

[34]   Yamamoto K, Horikita M, Tsuda F, Itoh K, Akahane Y, Yotsumoto S,
Okamoto H et al.(1995).Hepatitis B virus escape mutants:"pushing the
envelope" of chronic hepatitis B virus infection, *Hepatology*, 21(3): 884-
887.

[35]   Baumert TF, Barth H, Blum HE.(2005).Genetic variants of hepatitis B
virus and their clinical relevance. *Minerva Gastroenterol. Dietol*,
51(1):95-108.

[36]   Lin CL, Liao LY, Wang CS, et al. (2005). Basal core-promoter mutant of
hepatitis B virus and progression of liver disease in hepatitis B e antigen-
negative chronic hepatitis B. *Liver Int*,11(25): 564-570.

[37]   Chen BF, Liu CJ, Jow GM, et al.(2006).High prevalence and mapping of
pre-S deletion in hepatitis B virus carriers with progressive liver diseases.
Gastroenterology, 130(4):1153-1168.

[38]   Leon B, Taylor L, Vargas M, et al. (2005).HBx M130K and V131I (T-A)
mutations in HBV genotype F during a follow-up study in chronic
carriers. *J. Virol*, 2: 60.

[39]   Milich DR, Chen M, Schodel F, et al.(1997).Role of B cells in antigen
presentation of the hepatitis B core. *Proc. Natl. Acad. Sci. USA*,94(26):
14648-14653.

[40]   Mele A, Tancredi F, Romano L, Giuseppone A, Colucci M, Sangiuolo A,
Lecce R, Adamo B, Tosti ME, Taliani G, Zanetti AR.
(2001).Effectiveness of hepatitis B vaccination in babies born to hepatitis
B surface antigen-positive mothers in Italy. *J. Infect. Dis*, 184(7): 905-
908.

[41]   Zhong S, Chan JY, Yeo W, Tam JS, Johnson PJ.(1999).Hepatitis B
envelope protein mutants in human hepatocellular carcinoma tissues. *J.
Viral Hep*, 6(3):195-202.

[42]   He JW, Lu Q, Zhu QR, Duan SC,Wen YM.(1998).Mutations in the ′a′
determinant of hepatitis B surface antigen among Chinese infants
receiving active postexposure hepatitis B immunization. *Vaccine*,16(2-3):
170-173.

[43]   Kato J,Hasegawa K,Torii N,Yamauchi K, Hayashi N. (1996). A molecular analysis of viral persistence in surface antigen-negative chronic hepatitis B, *Hepatology*, 23(3):391-395.

[44]   Oon CJ, Chen WN. (1998).Current aspects of hepatitis B surface antigen mutants in Singapore. *J. Viral Hepatitis*, 5(Suppl 2): 17-23.

[45]   Schories M, Peters T, Rasenack J. (2000).Isolation, characterization and biological significance of hepatitis B virus mutants from serum of a patient with immunologically negative HBV infection. *J. Hepatol*, 33(5): 799-811.

[46]   Chirara MM, Chetsanga CJ.(1994).Variant of hepatitis B virus isolated in Zimbabwe. *J. Med. Virol*, 42(1):73–78.

[47]   Oon CJ, Lim GK,Ye Z, Goh KT, Tan KL, Yo SL, Hopes E, Harrison TJ, Zuckerman AJ.(1995).Molecular epidemiology of hepatitis B virus vaccine variants in Singapore. *Vaccine*, 13(8): 699–702.

[48]   Shields PL, Owsianka A, Carman WF, Boxall E,Hubscher SG, Shaw J, O'Donnell K, Elias E,Mutimer DJ.(1999).Selection of hepatitis B surface "escape" mutants during passive immune prophylaxis following liver transplantation: potential impact of genetic changes on polymerase protein function. *Gut*, 45(2):306-309.

[49]   Brind A, Jiang J, Samuel D, Gigou M, Feray C, Brechot C, Kremsdorf D. (1997).Evidence for selection of hepatitis B mutants after liver transplantation through peripheral blood mononuclear cell infection, *J. Hepatol*, 26(2): 228–235.

[50]   Protzer-Knolle U, Naumann U, Bartenschlager R, Berg T, Hopf U,Meyer zum Büschenfelde KH,Neuhaus P, Gerken G.(1998).Hepatitis B virus with antigenically altered hepatitis B surface antigen is selected by high-dose hepatitis B immune globulin after liver transplantation. *Hepatology*, 27(1):254-263.

[51]   Seddigh-Tonekaboni S, Lim WL, Young B, Hou JL, Waters J, Luo KX, Thomas HC, Karayiannis P.(2001).Hepatitis B surface antigen variants in vaccinees, blood donors and an interferon-treated patient. *J. Viral. Hepat*, 8(2): 154-158.

[52]   Oon CJ,Chen WN, Lim N, Koh S, Lim GK, Leong A, Tan GS.(1999). Hepatitis B virus variants with lamivudine-related mutations in the DNA polymerase and the 'a' epitope of the surface antigen are sensitive to ganciclovir. *Antiviral Researche*, 41(3): 113-118,

[53]   Sterneck M, Kalinina T, Günther S, Fischer L, Santantonio T, Greten H, Will H. (1998).Functional analysis of HBV genomes from patients with fulminant hepatitis. *Hepatology*, 28(5): 1390-1397.

[54]   Moraes MTB, Gomes SA, Niel C. (1996). Sequence analysis of pre–S/S gene of hepatitis B virus strains of genotypes A, D, and F isolated in Brazil. *Arch. Virol*, 141(9): 1767–1773.

[55]   Ho MS, Lu CF, Kuo J, Mau YC, Chao WH. (1995).A family cluster of an immune escape variant of hepatitis B virus infecting a mother and her two fully immunized children. *Clin. Diagn. Lab. Immunol*, 2(6):760–762,

[56]   Yamamoto K, Horikita M, Tsuda F, Itoh K, Akahane Y, Yotsumoto S, Okamoto H, Miyakawa Y, Mayumi M.(1994).Naturally occurring escape mutants of heptatitis B virus with various mutations in the S gene in carriers seropostive for antibody to hepatitis B surface antigen. *J. Virol*, 68(4):2671–2676.

[57]   Yoshida EM, Ramji A, Erb SR, Davis JE, Steinbrecher UP, Sherlock CH,Scudamore CH, Chung SW, Williams M,Gutfreund KS.(2000).De novo acute hepatitis B infection in a previously vaccinated liver transplant recipient due to a strain of HBV with a Met 133 Thr mutation in the "a"determinant, *Liver*, 20(5): 411-414.

[58]   Rodriguez-Frias F, Buti M, Jardi R, Vargas V, Quer J, Cotrina M, Martell M, Esteban R, Guardia J. (1999).Genetic alterations in the S gene of hepatitis B virus in patients with acute hepatitis B, chronic hepatitis B and hepatitis B liver cirrhosis before and after liver transplantation. *Liver*, 19(3): 177-182.

[59]   Chong-Jin O, Wei Ning C, Shiuan K, Gek Keow L.(1999). Identification of hepatitis B surface antigen variants with alterations outside the "a"determinant in immunized Singapore infants. *J. Infect. Dis*, 179(1): 259-263.

[60]   Kohno H, Inoue T, Tsuda F, Okamoto H, Akahane Y. (1996). Mutations in the envelope gene of hepatitis B virus variants co-occurring with antibody to surface antigen in sera from patients with chronic hapatitis B. *J. Gen. Virol*,77(pt8): 1825- 1831.

[61]   Fernholz D,Galle PR,Stemler M, Brunetto M, Bonino F, Will H.(1993).Infectious hepatitis B virus variant defective in pre-S2 protein expression in a chronic carrier. *Virology*, 194(1): 137–148.

[62]   Ahn S, Kramvis A, Kawai S, Spangenberg H, Li J, Kimbi G, Kew M, Wands J and Tong S.(2003).Sequence variation upstream of precore translation initiation codon reduces hepatitis B virus e antigen production. *Gastroenterology*,125(5): 1370-1378.

[63]   Okamoto H, Yotsumoto S, AkahaneY, Yamanaka T, Miyazaki Y, Sugai Y, Tsuda F, Tanaka T, Miyakawa Y, Mayumi M.(1990).Hepatitis B viruses with precore region defects prevail in persistently infected hosts along with seroconversion to the antibody against e antigen. *J. Virol*, 64(3): 1298-1303.

[64]   Omi S, Okamoto H,Tsuda F, Mayumi M.(1990).Defects in the precore region of hepatitis B virus DNA in a plasma pool from carriers seropositive for antibody against e antigen and with infectivity in chimpanzees. *J. Gastroenterol. Hepatol*, 5(6): 646-652.

[65]   Naoumov NV, Schneider R, Groetzinger T, Jung MC, Miska S, Pape R, Will H. (1992).Precore mutant hepatitis B virus infection and liver disease. *Gastroenterology*, 102(2): 538-543.

[66]   Inoue K, Yoshiba M, Sekiyama K,Okamoto H, Mayumi M. (1998).Clinical and molecular virological differences between fulminant hepatic failures following acute and chronic infection with hepatitis B virus. *J. Med. Virol*, 55(1): 35-41.

[67]   Hasegawa K, Huang J, Rogers SA, Blum HE, Liang TJ.(1994).Enhanced replication of a hepatitis B virus mutant associated with an epidemic of fulminant hepatitis. *J. Virol*, 68(3): 1651-1659.

[68]   Kosaka Y, Takase K, Kojima M,Shimizu M, Inoue K,Yoshiba M, Tanaka S, Akahane Y, Okamoto H, Tsuda F, et al.(1991). Fulminant hepatitis B: Induction by hepatitis B virus mutants defective in the precore region and incapable of encoding e antigen. *Gastroenterology*, 100(4): 1087-1094.

[69]   Liang TJ, Hasegawa K, Rimon N, Wands JR, Ben–Porath E.(1991).A hepatitis B virus mutant associated with an epidemic of fulminant hepatitis. *N. Engl. J. Med*, 324(24): 1705-1709.

[70]   Omata M, Ehata T, Yokosuka O, Hosoda K, Ohto M.(1991).Mutations in the precore region of hepatitis B virus DNA in patients with fulminant and severe hepatitis. *N. Engl. J. Med*, 324(24): 1699-1704.

[71]   Fujise K, Suzuki K, Naito Y, Niiya M, Ishikawa T, Takahashi H, Hoshina S, Saito A, Watanabe R. (1998). Hepatitis B virus variants in patients with acute hepatitis in whom various clinical forms develop. *Kansenshogaku Zasshi*, 72(1): 67-74.

[72]   Ito S, Nakazono K, Murasawa A, Mita Y, Hata K, Saito N,Kikuchi M, Yoshida K,Nakano M, Gejyo F. (2001). Development of fulminant hepatitis B(precore variant mutant type) after the discontinuation of low-dose methotrexate therapy in a rheumatoid arthritis patient. *Arthritis and Rheumatism*, 44(2): 339-342.

[73]   Zhong S, Chan JY, Yeo W, Tam JS, Johnson PJ.(2000).Frequent integration of precore/core mutants of hepatitis B virus in human hepatocellular carcinoma tissues. *J. Viral Hepatitis*, 7(2): 115-123.

[74]   Löhr HF, Weber W, Schlaak J, Goergen B, Meyer zum Büschenfelde KH,Gerken G.(1995). Proliferative response of CD4[+] T cells and hepatitis B virus clearance in chronic hepatitis with or without hepatitis B e-minus hepatitis B virus mutants. *Hepatology*, 22(1): 61–68.

[75]   Saellberg M, Ruden U,Wahren B, Noah M, Magnius LO. (1991). Human and murine B–cells recognize the HBeAg/beta (or HBe2) epitope as a linear determinant. *Mol. Immunol*, 28(7): 719–726.

[76]   Penna A, Bertoletti A, Cavalli A, Valli A, Missale G, Pilli M, Marchelli S, Giuberti T, Fowler P, Chisari FV, Fiaccadori F, Ferrari C.(1992).Fine specificity of the human T cell response to hepatitis B virus core antigen. *Arch. Virol. Suppl*, 4: 23–28.

[77]   Marinos G, Torre F, Günther S, Thomas MG, Will H, Williams R, Naoumov NV.(1996).Hepatitis B virus variants with core gene deletions in the evolution of chronic hepatitis B infection. *Gastroenterology*, 111(1): 183–192.

[78]   Günther S, Baginski S, Kissel H, Reinke P, Krüger DH, Will H, Meisel H. (1996).Accumulation and persistence of hepatitits B virus core gene deletion mutants in renal transplant patients are associated with end-stage liver disease. *Hepatology*, 24(4): 751–758.

[79]   Günther S, Li BC, Miska S, Krüger DH, Meisel H, Will H.(1995). A novel method for efficient amplification of whole hepatitis B virus genomes permits rapid functional analysis and reveals deletion mutants in immunosuppressed patients. *J. Virol*, 69(9): 5437–5444.

[80]   Preikschat P, Meisel H, Will H, Günther S. (1999). Hepatitis B virus genomes from long-term immunosuppressed virus carriers are modified by specific mutations in several regions. *J. Gen. Viro*, 80(pt10): 2685-2691.

[81]   Chang LJ, Hirsch RC, Ganem D, Varmus HE.(1990).Effects of insertional and point mutations on the functions of the duck hepatitis B virus polymerase. *J. Virol*, 64(11): 5553–5558.

[82]   Radziwill G, Tucker W, Schaller H.(1990). Mutational analysis of the hepatitis B virus P gene product: domain structure and RNase H activity. *J. Viro*, 64(2):613–620.

[83]   Fu L, Cheng YC. (1998). Role of additional mutations outside the YMDD motif of hepatitis B virus polymerase in L(-)SddC (3TC) resistance. *Biochem. Pharmacol*, 55(10): 1567–1572.

[84]   Melegari M, Scaglioni PP, Wands JR. (1998). Hepatitis B virus mutants associated with 3TC and famciclovir administration are replication defective. *Hepatology*, 27(2): 628–633.

[85]   Chen Y, Robinson WS, Marion PL. (1992).Naturally occurring point mutation in the C terminus of the polymerase gene prevents duck hepatitis B virus RNA packaging. *J. Virol*, 66(2): 1282–1287.

[86]   Uchida T, Gotoh K, Shikata T. (1995). Complete nucleotide sequences and the characteristics of two hepatitis B virus mutants causing serologically negative acute or chronic hepatitis B. *J. Med. Virol* , 45(3): 247–252.

[87]   Uchida T, Shimojima M, Gotoh K, Shikata T, Tanaka E, Kiyosawa K. (1994). "Silent" hepatitis B virus mutants are responsible for non-A, non-B, non-C, non-D, non-E hepatitis. *Microbiol. Immunol* , 38(4):281–285.

[88]   Hsia CC, Nakashima Y, Tabor E. (1997).Deletion mutants of the hepatitis B virus X gene in human hepatocellular carcinoma. *Biochem. Biophys. Res. Commun*, 241(3): 726–729.

[89]   Feitelson M, Lega L, Guo J, Resti M, Rossi ME, Azzari C, Blumberg BS, Vierucci A.(1994).Pathogenesis of posttransfusion viral hepatitis in children with b–thalassemia. *Hepatology*, 19(3): 558–568.

[90]   Feitelson MA, Duan LX, Guo J, Horiike N, McIntyre G, Blumberg BS, Thomas HC, Carman W.(1995). Precore and X region mutants in hepatitis B virus infections among renal dialysis patients. *J. Viral. Hepat*, 2(1): 19-31.

[91]   Rizzetto M, Canese MG, Arico S, et al. (1977).Immunofluorescence detection of new antigen-antibody system (delta/anti-delta) associated to hepatitis B virus in liver and in serum of HBsAg carriers. *Gut*,18(12):997-1003.

[92]   Rizzetto M,Verme G.(1985).Delta hepatitis-present status. *J. Hepatol*,1(2) :187-93.

[93]   Govindarajan S, Chin KP, Redeker AG, Peters RI.(1984).Fulminant B viral hepatitis: role of delta agent. *Gastroenterology*, 86(6):1417-20.

[94]   Smedile A, Farci P, Verme G, et al. (1982). Influence of delta infection on severity of hepatitis B. *Lancet*, 2(8305):945-947.

[95]   Leung N. (2005).HBV and liver cancer. Med. *J. Malaysia*, 60 (Suppl B):63-66.

[96]   Chen SL, Morgan TR. (2006).The natural history of hepatitis C virus (HCV) infection. *In. J. Med. Sci*, 3(2):7-52.

[97]   Brechot C, Gozuacik D, Murakami Y, et al.(2000).Molecular bases for the development of hepatitis B virus (HBV)-related hepatocellular carcinoma (HCC). *Semin. Cancer Biol*, 10(3), 211-31.

[98]   Monto A, Wright TL.(2001).The epidemiology and prevention of hepatocellular carcinoma. *Semin. Oncol*, 28(5):441-9.

[99]   Bukhtiari N, Hussain T, Iqbal M, et al. (2003).Hepatitis B and C single and co-infection in chronic liver disease and their effect on the disease pattern. *J. Pak. Med. Assoc*, 2003, 53(4): 136-140.

[100]   Fattovich G, Stroffolini T, Zagni I, et al. (2004). Hepatocellular carcinoma in cirrhosis: incidence and risk factors. *Gastroenterology*, 127(5Suppl1): S35-50.

[101]   Park JS, Saraf N, Dieterich DT.(2006).HBV plus HCV, HCV plus HIV, HBV plus HIV. *Curr. Gastroenterol. Rep*, 8(1): 67-74.

[102]   Michielsen PP, Francque SM, van Dongen JL.(2005).Viral hepatitis and hepatocellular carcinoma. *World J. Surg. Oncol*, 3: 27.

[103]   Schuttler CG , Fiedler N, Schmidt K, et al.(2002).Suppression of hepatitis B virus enhancer 1 and 2 by hepatitis C virus core protein . *J. Hepatol*, 37(6):855-862.

[104]   Chen SY, Kao CF, Chen CM, et al. (2003).Mechanisms for inhibition of hepatitis B virus gene expression and replication by hepatitis C virus core protein. *J. Biol. Chem*, 278(1):591-607.

[105]   Dumoulin FL, von dem Bussche A, Li J, et al. (2003). Hepatitis C virus NS2 protein inhibits gene expression from different cellular and viral promoters in hepatic and nonhepatic cell lines. *Virology*, 305(2):260-266.

[106]   Carr A, Cooper DA.(1997).Restoration of immunity to chronic hepatitis B infection in HIV-infected patient on protease inhibitor. *Lancet*, 349:995-996.

[107]   Schnittman SM, Pierce PF. (1996). Potential role of lamivudine (3TC) in the clearance of chronic hepatitis B virus infection in a patient coinfected with human immunodeficiency virus type 1. *Clin. Infect. Dis*, 23(3):638-639.

[108]   Sherman M. (2006).Optimizing management strategies in special patient populations. *Am. J. Gastroenterol*, 101 (Suppl1):S26-31.

[109]   Bruno R, Puoti M, Sacchi P, et al. (2006).Management of hepatocellular carcinoma in human immunodeficiency virus-infected patients. *J. Hepatol*, 44(Suppl): S146-150.

[110]   Lok ASF, Chung H-T, Liu VWS, Ma OCK. (1993). Long-term follow-up of chronic hepatitis B patients treated with interferon alfa. *Gastroenterology*, 105(6):1833-1838.

[111]   Lok ASF, Ma OCK, Lau JYN.(1991).Interferon alfa therapy in patients with chronic hepatitis B virus infection: effects on hepatitis B virus DNA in the liver. *Gastroenterology*, 100(3):756-761.

[112]   McMahon BJ, Alberts SR, Wainwright RB et al. (1990).Hepatitis B-related sequelae. Prospective study in 1400 hepatitis B surface antigen-positive Alaska Native carriers. *Arch. Intern. Med*, 150(5):1051-1054.

[113]   Beasley RP.(1988).Hepatitis B virus.The major etiology of hepatocellular carcinoma. Cancer, 61(10):1942-1956.

[114]   Yang HI, Lu SN, et al.(2002).Hepatitis B e antigen and the risk of hepatocellular carcinoma. *N. Engl. J. Med*, 347(3):168-174.

[115]   Hino O. (2005).Intentional delay of human hepatocarcinogenesis due to suppression of chronic hepatitis. *Intervirology*, 48(1):6-9.

[116]   Chan HL, Sung JJ.(2006).Hepatocellular carcinoma and hepatitis B virus. *Semin. Liver Dis*, 26(2), 153-161.

[117]   Hino O, Kajino K, Umeda T, et al. (2002). Understanding the hypercarcinogenic state in chronic hepatitis: a clue to the prevention of human hepatocellular carcinoma. *J. Gastroenterol*, 37(11):883-7.

[118]   Blum HE. (2002).Molecular targets for prevention of hepatocellular carcinoma. *Dig. Dis*, 20(1), 81-90.

[119]   Cougot D, Neuveut C, Buendia MA.(2005). HBV induced carcinogenesis. *J. Clin. Virol*, 34 (Suppl 1):S75-78.

[120]   Trere D, Borzio M, Morabito A, et al. (2003). Nucleolar hypertrophy correlates with hepatocellular carcinoma development in cirrhosis due to HBV infection. *Hepatology*, 37(1):72-78.

[121]   D'Assoro AB, Lingle WL, Salisbury JL et al. (2002).Centrosome amplification and the development of cancer. *Oncogene*, 21(40):6146–6153.

[122] Yun C, Cho H, Kim SJ, et al. (2004). Mitotic aberration coupled with centrosome amplification is induced by hepatitis B virus X oncoprotein via the Ras-mitogen-activated protein/extracellular signal-regulated kinase-mitogen- activated protein pathway. *Mol. Cancer Res*, 2(3), 159–169.

[123] Peng Z, Zhang Y, Gu W, et al. (2005).Integration of the hepatitis B virus X fragment in hepatocellular carcinoma and its effects on the expression of multiple molecules: a key to the cell cycle and apoptosis. *Int. J. Oncol*, 26(2): 467-473.

[124] Dominguez-Malagon H, Gaytan-Graham S. (2001).Hepatocellular carcinoma: an update. *Ultrastruct. Pathol*, 25:497-516.

[125] Szabo E, Paska C, Kaposi Novak P, Schaff Z, Kiss A.(2004). Similarities and differences in hepatitis B and C virus induced hepatocarcinogenesis. *Pathol. Oncol. Res.* 10(1): 5-11.

[126] Dienes HP, Gerken G, Goergen B, Heermann K, Gerlich W, Meyer zum, Buschenfelde KH.(1995).Analysis of the precore DNA sequence and detection of precore antigen in liver specimens from patients with anti-hepatitis B e–positive chronic hepatitis. *Hepatology*, 21: 1–7.

[127] Wang XH, Wang PL. (2003).Relationship between mutation on precore region of integrated HBV DNA and p53 gene mutation in hepatocellular carcinoma. *Ai. Zheng*, 22:715-8.

[128] Hwang GY, Lin CY, Huang LM, Wang YH, Wang JC, Hsu CT, et al. (2003).Detection of the hepatitis B virus X protein (HBx) antigen and anti-HBx antibodies in cases of human hepatocellular carcinoma. *J. Clin. Microbiol*, 41(12): 5598-5603.

[129] Zhang X, Dong N, Zhang H, You J, Wang H and Ye LH.(2005).Effects of hepatitis B virus X protein on hTERT expression and activity in hepatoma cells. *J. Lab. Clin. Med*, 145(2):98-104.

[130] Levrero M, Stemler M, Pasquinelli C, Alberti A, Jean-Jean O, Franco A,et al. (1991).Significance of anti-HBx antibodies in hepatitis B virus infection. *Hepatology*, 13(1):143-149.

[131] Zhang X, Zhang H, Ye L. (2006).Effects of hepatitis B virus X protein on the development of liver cancer. *J. Lab. Clin. Med*, 147:58-66.

[132] Kim JW, Shim JH, Park JW, et al. (2005).Development of PCR-ELISA for the detection of hepatitis B virus x gene expression and clinical application. *J. Clin. Lab. Anal*, 19:139-45.

[133] Ou DP, Tao YM, Chang ZG, et al.(2006).Hepatocellular carcinoma cells containing hepatitis B virus X protein have enhanced invasive potential conditionally. *Dig. Liver Dis*, 38:262-267.

[134] Han J, Yoo HY, Choi BH, Rho HM.(2000).Selective transcriptional regulations in the human liver cell by hepatitis B viral X protein. *Bioc. Biop. Res. Comm*, 272(2): 525-530.

[135] Gottlob K, Fulco M, Levrero M, Graessmann A. (1998). The Hepatitis B virus HBx protein inhibits caspase 3 activity. *J. Biol. Chem*, 273: 33347 - 33353.

[136] Chami M, Ferrari D, Nicotera P, Paterlini-Bréchot P, Rizzuto R.(2003). Caspase-dependent alterations of Ca^{2+} signaling in the induction of apoptosis by hepatitis B virus X protein. *J. Biol. Chem*, 278(34): 31745-31755.

[137] Kim WH, Hong F, Jaruga B, et al. (2005).Hepatitis B virus X protein sensitizes primary mouse hepatocytes to ethanol- and TNF-alpha-induced apoptosis by a caspase-3-dependent mechanism. *Cell Mol. Immunol*, 2:40-48.

[138] Li D, Chen X, Zhang W. (2003). The inhibition of apoptosis of hepatoma cells induced by HBx is mediated by up-regulation of survivin expression. *J. Huazhong. Univ. Sci. Technolog. Med. Sci*, 23(4): 383-386.

[139] Zhang X, Dong N, Yin L, Cai N, Ma H, You J, et al. (2005). Hepatitis B virus X protein up-regulates survivin expression in hepatoma tissues. *J. Med. Virol*,77: 374-381.

[140] Marusawa H, Matsuzawa S, Welsh K, Zou H, Armstrong R, Tamm I, et al. (2003). HBXIP functions as a cofactor of survivin in apoptosis suppression. *EMBO J*, 22: 2729 - 2740.

[141] Kucharczak J, Simmons MJ, Fan Y, Gelinas C. (2003).To be, or not to be: NF-kappaB is the answer--role of Rel/NF-kappaB in the regulation of apoptosis. *Oncogene*, 22(56): 8961-8982.

[142] Chang F, Steelman LS, Shelton JG, Lee JT, Navolanic PM, Blalock WL, et al. (2003).Regulation of cell cycle progression and apoptosis by the Ras/Raf/MEK/ERK pathway. *Int. J. Oncol*, 22(3): 469-480.

[143] Sheikh MS, Fornace AJ Jr. (2000).Role of p53 family members in apoptosis. *J. Cell Physiol*, 182(2): 171-181.

[144] Shen Y, White E. (2001).p53-dependent apoptosis pathways. *Adv. Cancer Res*, 82: 55-84.

[145] Bates S, Vousden KH.(1999).Mechanisms of p53-mediated apoptosis. *Cell Mol. Life Sci*, 55(1): 28-37.

[146] Hanahan D and Weinberg RA. (2000).The Hallmarks of Cancer. *Cell*, 100: 57–70.

[147] Qadri I, Ferrari ME, Siddiqui A. (1996). The hepatitis B virus transactivator protein, HBx, interacts with single-stranded DNA (ss-DNA).Biochemical characterizations of the HBx-ssDNA interactions. *J. Biol. Chem*, 271(26): 15443–15450.

[148] Haviv I, Vaizel D, Shaul Y. (1996). pX the HBV-encoded coactivator, interacts with components of the transcription machinery and stimulates transcription in a TAF-independent manner. *EMBO J*, 15(13): 3413–3420.

[149] Colgrove R, Simon G, and Ganem D.(1989).Transcriptional activation of homologous and heterologous genes by the hepatitis B virus X gene product in cells permissive for viral replication. *J. Virol*, 63:4019–4026.

[150] Seto E, Mitchell PJ, Yen TS. (1990). Transactivation by the hepatitis B virus X protein depends on AP-2 and other transcription factors. *Nature*, 344(6261): 72–74.

[151] Lucito R, Schneider RJ. (1992). Hepatitis B virus X protein activates transcription factor NF-kappa B without a requirement for protein kinase C. *J. Virol*, 66(2): 983–991.

[152] Lee JS, Heo J, Libbrecht L, et al. (2006). A novel prognostic subtype of human hepatocellular carcinoma derived from hepatic progenitor cells. *Nat. Med*, 12:410-416.

[153] Tanaka Y, Kanai F, Ichimura T, et al.(2006). The hepatitis B virus X protein enhances AP-1 activation through interaction with Jab1. *Oncogene*, 25:633-42.

[154] Andrisani OM, Barnabas S.(1999).The transcriptional function of the hepatitis B virus X protein and its role in hepatocarcinogenesis. *Int. J. Oncol*, 15(2):373–379.

[155] Wentz MJ, Becker SA, Slagle BL.(2000).Dissociation of DDB1-binding and transactivation properties of the hepatitis B virus X protein. *Virus Res*, 68(1): 87–92.

[156] Chirillo P, Falco M, Puri PL, Artini M, Balsano C, Levrero M. (1996). Hepatitis B virus pX activates NF-kappa B-dependent transcription through a Raf-independent pathway. *J.Virol*, 70(1): 641–646.

[157] Menzo S, Clementi M, Alfani E, Bagnarelli P, Iacovacci S, Manzin A. (1993).Trans-activation of epidermal growth factor receptor gene by the hepatitis B virus X-gene product. *Virology*, 196(2): 878–882.

[158]   Wang C, Wang W, Lu H.(1997).Immunohistochemical study of hepatitis C virus core antigen and HBxAg in liver cirrhosis and hepatocellular carcinoma tissues. *Chung Hua Chung Liu Tsa Chih*, 19(2):85–88.

[159]   Henkler F, Lopes AR, Jones M, Koshy R.(1998).Erk-independent partial activation of AP-1 sites by the hepatitis B virus HBx protein. *J. Gen. Virol*, 79: 2737–2742.

[160]   Benn J, Schneider RJ. (1995). Hepatitis B virus HBx protein deregulates cell cycle checkpoint controls. *Proc. Natl. Acad. Sci. USA* , 92:11215-11219.

[161]   Mansour SJ, Matten WT, Hermann AS, Candia JM, Rong S, Fukasawa K, et al. (1994).Transformation of mammalian cells by constitutively active MAP kinase. *Science*, 265:966-970.

[162]   Choi CY, Choi BH, Park GT, Rho HM. (1997). Activating transcription factor 2(ATF2) down-regulates hepatitis B virus X promoter activity by the competition for the activating protein 1 binding site and the formation of the ATF2-Jun heterodimer. *J. Biol. Chem*, 272: 16934-16939.

[163]   Tarn C, Zou L, Hullinger RL, Andrisani OM. (2002). Hepatitis B virus X protein activates the p38 mitogen-activated protein kinase pathway in dedifferentiated hepatocytes. *J. Virol*,76: 9763 - 9772.

[164]   Lee YI, Park SK, Do SI, Lee YI. (2001).The Hepatitis B virus-X protein activates a phosphatidylinositol 3-kinase-dependent survival signaling cascade. *J. Biol. Chem*, 276: 16969 - 16977.

[165]   Klein NP, Bouchard MJ, Wang LH, Kobarg C, Schneider RJ.(1999).Src kinases involved in hepatitis B virus replication. *EMBO J*, 18(18):5019–5027.

[166]   Lee YH, Yun Y. (1998). HBx protein of hepatitis B virus activates Jak1-STAT signaling. *J. Biol. Chem*, 273(39):25510–25515.

[167]   Waris G, Huh KW, Siddiqui A. (2001).Mitochondrially Associated Hepatitis B Virus X Protein Constitutively Activates Transcription Factors STAT-3 and NF-κB via Oxidative Stress. *Mol. Cell Biol*, 21:7721 – 7730 .

[168]   Ruff-Jamison S, Chen K, Cohen S. (1995). Epidermal growth factor induces the tyrosine phosphorylation -and nuclear translocation of Stat 5 in mouse liver. *Proc. Natl. Acad. Sci*, 92: 4215-4218.

[169]   Cressman DE, Diamond RH, Taub R.(1995).Rapid activation of the Stat3 transcription complex in liver regeneration. *Hepatology* , 5: 1443-1449.

[170] Feitelson MA, Zhu M, Duan L-X, London WT. (1993). Hepatitis B X antigen and p53 are associated in vitro and in liver tissues from patients with primary hepatocellular carcinoma. *Oncogene*, 8: 1109-1117.

[171] Lee SH, Park SG, Lim SO, et al. (2005). The hepatitis B virus X protein up-regulates lymphotoxin alpha expression in hepatocytes. *Biochim. Biophys. Acta*, 1741:75-84.

[172] Pan J, Duan LX, Sun BS, Feitelson MA. (2001). Hepatitis B virus X protein protects against anti-Fas-mediated apoptosis in human liver cells by inducing NF-κB. *J. Gen. Virol*, 82: 171 – 182.

[173] Yun C, Um HR, Jin YH, Wang JH, Lee MO, Park S, et al. (2002). NF-kappaB activation by hepatitis B virus X (HBx) protein shifts the cellular fate toward survival. *Cancer Lett*, 184(1): 97-104.

[174] Wang T, Wang Y, Wu MC, Guan XY, Yin ZF. (2004).Activating mechanism of transcriptor NF-kappaB regulated by hepatitis B virus X protein in hepatocellular carcinoma. *World J. Gastroenterol*, 10(3):356-360.

[175] Ryu WS. (2003).Molecular aspects of hepatitis B viral infection and the viral carcinogenesis. *J. Biochem. Mol. Biol*, 36:138-43.

[176] Lee TH, Tai DI, Cheng CJ, et al. Enhanced nuclear factor-kappa B-associated Wnt-1 expression in hepatitis B- and C-related hepatocarcinogenesis: identification by functional proteomics. *J. Biomed. Sci*, 2006; 13(1),27-39.

[177] Birrer RB, Birrer D, and Klavins JV.(2003).Hepatocellular carcinoma and hepatitis virus. *Ann. Clin. Lab. Sci*, 33(1): 39-54.

[178] Koike K, Moriya K, Yotsuyanagi H, Iino S, Kurokawa K.(1994).Induction of cell cycle progression by hepatitis B virus HBx gene expression in quiescent mouse fibroblasts. *J. Clin. Invest*, 94(1): 44-49.

[179] Wu BK, Li CC, Chen HJ, et al. (2006).Blocking of G1/S transition and cell death in the regenerating liver of Hepatitis B virus X protein transgenic mice. *Biochem. Biophys. Res. Commun*, 340:916-28.

[180] Shih WL, Kuo ML, Chuang SE, Cheng AL, Doong SL. (2000). Hepatitis B virus X protein inhibits transforming growth factor-β-induced apoptosis through the activation of phosphatidylinositol 3-kinase pathway. *J. Biol. Chem*, 275: 25858-25864.

[181] Park SG, Chung C, Kang H, Kim JY, Jung G.(2006).Up-regulation of
       cyclin D1 by HBx is mediated by NF-kappa B2/BCL3 complex through
       kappa B site of cyclin D1 promoter. *J. Biol. Chem,.* 281(42):31770-
       31777.

[182] Poole JC, Andrews LG, Tollefsbol TO.(2001).Activity, function, and gene
       regulation of the catalytic subunit of telomerase (hTERT). *Gene,* 269: 1-
       12.

[183] Horikawa I, Barrett JC.(2001).Cis-Activation of the human telomerase
       gene (hTERT) by the hepatitis B virus genome. *J. Natl. Cancer Inst,* 93:
       1171-1173.

[184] Wang WL, Gu GY, Hu M. (1998).Expression and significance of HBV
       genes   and   their   antigens   in   human   primary   intrahepatic
       cholangiocarcinoma. *World J. Gastroenterol,* 4: 392-396.

[185] Dubiel W, Ferrell K, Pratt G, Reichsteiner M.(1992).Subunit 4 of the 26 S
       protease is a member of a novel eukaryotic ATPase family. *J. Biol. Chem,*
       267: 22699–22702.

[186] Lee AT, Ren J, Wong ET, et al. (2005). The hepatitis B virus X protein
       sensitizes HepG2 cells to UV light-induced DNA damage. *J. Biol. Chem,*
       280:33525-35.

[187] Shiyanov P, Hayes SA, Donepudi M, Nichols AF, Linn S, Slagle BL, et
       al. (1999). The naturally occurring mutants of DDB are impaired in
       stimulating nuclear import of the p125 subunit and E2F1-activated
       transcription. *Mol. Cell Biol,* 19:4935-4943.

[188] Abramic M, Levine AS, Protic M. (1991).Purification of an ultraviolet-
       inducible, damage-specific DNA-binding protein from primate cells. *J.
       Biol. Chem,* 266:22493-22500.

[189] Sanz-Cameno P, Martin-Vilchez S, Lara-Pezzi E, et al. (2006). Hepatitis
       B virus promotes angiopoietin-2 expression in liver tissue: role of HBV x
       protein. *Am. J. Pathol,* 169:1215-1222.

[190] Bergametti F, Sitterlin D, Transy C. (2002). Turnover of Hepatitis B Virus
       X Protein Is Regulated by Damaged DNA-Binding Complex. *J. Virol,* 76:
       6495-6501.

[191] Benn J, Schneider RJ. (1994). Hepatitis B virus HBx protein activates
       Ras-GTP complex formation and establishes a Ras, Raf, MAP kinase
       signaling cascade. *Proc. Natl. Acad. Sci. USA,* 91:10350–10354.

[192] Lin GY, Paterson RG, Richardson CD, Lamb RA.(1998).The V protein of the paramyxovirus SV5 interacts with damage-specific DNA binding protein. *Virology*, 249:189-200.

[193] Kwee L, Lucito R, Aufiero B, Schneider RJ. (1992). Alternate translation initiation on hepatitis B virus X mRNA produces multiple polypeptides that differentially transactivate class II and III promoters. *J. Virol*, 66:4382–4389.

[194] Wang XW, Forrester K, Yeh H, et al. (1994) Hepatitis B virus X protein inhibits p53 sequence-specific DNA binding, transcriptional activity, and association with transcription factor ERCC3. *Proc. Natl. Acad. Sci .USA*, 91(6):2230-2234.

[195] Cedrone A, Covino M, Caturelli E, et al.(2000).Utility of alpha-fetoprotein (AFP) in the screening of patients with virus-related chronic liver disease: does different viral etiology influence AFP levels in HCC?A study in 350 western patients. *Hepatogastroenterology*, 47:1654-8.

[196] Barnabas S, Hai T, Andrisani OM.(1997). The hepatitis B virus X protein enhances the DNA-binding potential and transcription efficacy of bZip transcription factors. *J. Biol. Chem*, 272:20684–20690.

[197] Qadri I, Conaway JW, Conaway RC, Schaack J, Siddiqui A. (1996). Hepatitis B virus transactivator protein, HBx, associates with the components of TFIIH and stimulates the DNA helicase activity of TFIIH. *Proc. Natl. Acad. Sci*, 93: 10578-10583.

[198] Lin Y, Nomura T, Cheong JH, Dorjsuren D, Iida K, Murakami S.(1997).Hepatitis B virus X protein is a transcriptional modulator that communicates with transcription factor IIB and the RNA polymerase II subunit 5. *J. Biol. Chem*, 272:7132-7139.

[199] Rahmani Z, Huh KW, Lasher R, Siddiqui A.(2000). Hepatitis B virus X protein colocalizes to mitochondria with a human voltage-dependent anion channel, HVDAC3, and alters its transmembrane potential. *J. Virol*, 74: 2840-2846.

[200] Jaitovich-Groisman I, Benlimame N, Slagle BL, Perez MH, Alpert L, Song DJ, et al. (2001).Transcriptional regulation of the TFIIH transcription repair components XPB and XPD by the hepatitis B virus x protein in liver cells and transgenic liver tissue. *J. Biol. Chem*, 276(17): 14124-14132.

[201] Shirakata Y, Koike K. (2003). Hepatitis B virus X protein induces cell death by causing loss of mitochondrial membrane potential. *J. Biol. Chem*, 278: 22071-22078.

[202] Fields S, Song O-K.(1989).A novel genetic system to detect protein-protein interactions. *Nature*, 340: 245–246.

[203] Gyuris J, Golemis E, Chertkov H, Brent R. (1993). Cdi1, a human G1 and S phase protein phosphatase that associates with Cdk2. *Cell* , 75: 791–803.

[204] Dubiel W, Ferrell K, Rechsteiner M. (1995).Subunits of the regulatory complex of the 26S protease. *Mol. Biol. Rep*, 21: 27–34.

[205] Coux O, Tanaka K, Goldberg AL. (1996).Structure and functions of the 20S and 26S proteasomes. *Annu. Rev. Biochem*, 65: 801–847.

[206] Zhang ZS, Torii N, Furusaka A, Malayaman N, Hu ZY, Liang TJ.(2000).Structural and functional characterization of interaction between hepatitis B virus X protein and the proteasome complex. *J. Biol. Chem*, 275: 15157-15165.

[207] Tanaka Y, Kanai F, Kawakami T, Tateishi K, Ijichi H, Kawabe T, et al. (2004). Interaction of the hepatitis B virus X protein (HBx) with heat shock protein 60 enhances HBx-mediated apoptosis. *Biochem. Biophys. Res. Commun* , 318(2): 461-469.

[208] Zhang SM, Sun DC, Lou S, Bo XC, Lu Z, Qian XH, Wang SQ. (2005).HBx protein of hepatitis B virus (HBV) can form complex with mitochondrial HSP60 and HSP70. *Arch. Virol*, 150:1579-90.

[209] Sohn SY, Kim JH, Baek KW, et al. (2006). Turnover of hepatitis B virus X protein is facilitated by Hdj1, a human Hsp40/DnaJ protein. *Biochem. Biophys. Res. Commun*, 347:764-8.

[210] Sohn SY, Kim SB, Kim J, et al. (2006).Negative regulation of hepatitis B virus replication by cellular Hsp40/DnaJ proteins through destabilization of viral core and X proteins. *J. Gen. Virol*, 87:1883-1891

[211] Okuda K. (2000).Hepatocellular carcinoma. *J. Hepatol* , 32: 225-37.

[212] Tralhao JG, Roudier J, Morosan S et al. (2002).Paracrine in vivo inhibitory effects of hepatitis B virus X protein (HBx) on liver cell proliferation: An alternative mechanism of HBx-related pathogenesis. *Proc. Natl. Acad. Sci. USA.*,99(10):6991–6996.

[213] Sakamoto Y, Mafune K, Mori M, et al. (2000).Overexpression of MMP-9 correlates with growth of small hepatocellular carcinoma. *Int. J. Oncol*, 17:237–243.

[214] Kwon OS, Lim do Y, Kwon KA, et al. (2003).Clinical usefulness of plasma activities of gelatinase (matrix metalloproteinase-2 and 9) in chronic liver disease. *Taehan Kan Hakhoe Chi*, 9: 222-30.

[215] Chung TW, Lee YC, Kim CH. (2004). Hepatitis B viral HBx induces matrix metalloproteinase-9 gene expression through activation of ERK and PI-3K/AKT pathways: involvement of invasive potential. *FASEB J,* 18(10):1123-5.

[216] Chung TW, Kim JR, Suh JI, et al. (2004).Correlation between plasma levels of matrix metalloproteinase (MMP)-9 /MMP-2 ratio and alpha-fetoproteins in chronic hepatitis carrying hepatitis B virus. *J. Gastroenterol. Hepatol*, 19:565-71.

[217] Yu FL, Liu HJ, Lee JW, et al. (2005). Hepatitis B virus X protein promotes cell migration by inducing matrix metalloproteinase-3. *J. Hepatol*, 42:520-7.

[218] Lee JO, Kwun HJ, Jung JK, et al. (2005). Hepatitis B virus X protein represses E-cadherin expression via activation of DNA methyltransferase 1. *Oncogene*, 24:6617-25.

[219] Han J, Ding L, Yuan B, et al. (2006). Hepatitis B virus X protein and the estrogen receptor variant lacking exon 5 inhibit estrogen receptor signaling in hepatoma cells. *Nucleic Acids Res,* 34:3095-106.

[220] Zhang S, Lin R, Zhou Z, et al. (2006). Macrophage migration inhibitory factor interacts with HBx and inhibits its apoptotic activity. *Biochem. Biophys. Res. Commun*, 342:671-9.

[221] Cui F, Wang Y, Wang J, et al. (2006).The up-regulation of proteasome subunits and lysosomal proteases in hepatocellular carcinomas of the HBx gene knockin transgenic mice. *Proteomics*, 6:498-504.

[222] Sells MA, Chen ML, Acs G. (1987). Production of hepatitis B virus particles in Hep G2 cells transfected with cloned hepatitis B virus DNA. *Proceedings of the National Academy of Sciences, USA*, 84:1005–1009.

[223] Korba BE, Gerin JL.(1992).Use of a standardized cell culture assay to assess activities of nucleoside analogs against hepatitis B virus replication. *Antiviral. Research*, 19:55–70.

[224] Ladner SK, Otto MJ, Barker CS, Zaifert K,Wang GH, Guo JT, Seeger C , King RW. (1997). Inducible expression of human hepatitis B virus (HBV) in stably transfected hepatoblastoma cells: a novel system for screening potential inhibitors of HBV replication. *Antimicrobial Agents and Chemotherapy*, 41:1715–1720.

[225] Ladner SK, Miller TJ, Otto MJ, King RW. (1998).The hepatitis B virus M539V polymerase variation responsible for 3TC resistance also confers cross-resistance to other nucleoside analogues. *Antiviral Chemistry and Chemotherapy*, 9:65–72.

[226] Lin E, Luscombe C, Colledge D,Wang YY and Locarnini S . (1998).
       Long-term therapy with guanine nucleoside analog penciclovir controls
       chronic duck hepatitis B virus infection in vivo. *Antimicrobial Agents and
       Chemotherapy*, 42:2132–2137.

[227] Lander HJ, Holland PV, Alter, HJ, Chanock RM, Purcell
       RH.(1972).Antibody to hepatitis-associated antigen.frequency and pattern
       of response as detected by radioimmunoprecipitation. *JAMA*,
       220(8):1079–1082.

[228] MacDonald DM, Holmes EC, Lewis JC, Simmonds P.(2000).Detection of
       hepatitis B virus infection in wild-born chimpanzees(Pan troglodytes
       verus): phylogenetic relationships with human and other primate
       genotypes. *J. Virol*, 74(9):4253–4257.

[229] Takahashi K, Brotman B, Usuda S, Mishiro S, Prince AM. (2000).
       Fullgenome sequence analyses of hepatitis B virus (HBV) strains
       recovered from chimpanzees infected in the wild: implications for an
       origin of HBV. *Virology*, 267(1):58–64.

[230] Hu X, Margolis HS, Purcell RH, Ebert J, Robertson BH.(2000).
       Identification of hepatitis B virus indigenous to chimpanzees. *Proc. Natl.
       Acad. Sci. USA*, 97(4):1661–1664.

[231] Yan RQ, Su JJ, Huang DR, Gan YC, Yang C, Huang GH.(1996). Human
       hepatitis B virus and hepatocellular carcinoma. I. Experimental infection
       of tree shrews with hepatitis B virus. *J. Cancer Res. Clin. Oncol*, 122(5):
       283–288.

[232] Walter E, Keist R, Niederost B, Pult I, Blum HE.(1996).Hepatitis B virus
       infection of tupaia hepatocytes in vitro and in vivo. *Hepatology*, 24(1): 1–
       5.

[233] Glebe D, Aliakbari M, Krass P, Knoop EV, Valerius KP, Gerlich WH.(
       2003). Pre-S1 antigen-dependent infection of Tupaia hepatocyte cultures
       with human hepatitis B virus. *J. Virol*, 77(17):9511–9521.

[234] Kock J, Nassal M, MacNelly S, Baumert TF, Blum HE, von Weizsacker
       F. (2001). Efficient infection of primary tupaia hepatocytes with purified
       human and woolly monkey hepatitis B virus. *J. Virol*, 75(11):5084–5089.

[235] Li Y, Su JJ, Qin LL, Yang C, Ban KC, Yan RQ.(1999).Synergistic effect
       of hepatitis B virus and aflatoxin B1 in hepatocarcinogenesis in tree
       shrews. *Ann. Acad. Med. Singapore*, 28(1): 67–71.

[236] Yan RQ, Su JJ, Huang DR, Gan YC, Yang C, Huang GH.(1996).Human hepatitis B virus and hepatocellular carcinoma. II. Experimental induction of hepatocellular carcinoma in tree shrews exposed to hepatitis B virus and aflatoxin B1. *J. Cancer Res. Clin. Oncol*, 122(5):289–295.

[237] Zhai W, Gabor G, Acs G and Paronetto F.(1990).A nude mouse model for the in vivo production of hepatitis B virus. *Gastroenterology*, 98:470–477.

[238] Yao Z, Zhou Y, Feng X, Chen C and Guo J. (1996).In vivo inhibition of hepatitis B viral gene expression by antisense phosphorothioate oligodeoxynucleotides in athymic nude mice. *Journal of Viral Hepatology*, 3:19–22.

[239] Marion PL, Oshiro LS, Regnery DC, Scullard GH, Robinson WS.(1980).A virus in Beechey ground squirrels that is related to hepatitis B virus of humans. *Proc. Natl. Acad. Sci. USA* , 77(5):2941–2945.

[240] Mason WS, Seal G, Summers J. (1980). Virus of Pekin ducks with structural and biological relatedness to human hepatitis B virus. *J. Virol*, 36(3): 829–836.

[241] Summers J, Smolec JM, Snyder R. (1978). A virus similar to human hepatitis B virus associated with hepatitis and hepatoma in woodchucks. *Proc. Natl. Acad. Sci. USA* , 75(9):4533–4537.

[242] Summers J. (1981). Three recently described animal virus models for human hepatitis B virus. *Hepatology*, 1(2):179–183.

[243] Gerin JL, Cote PJ, Korba BE, Tennant BC.(1989).Hepadnavirusinduced liver cancer in woodchucks. *Cancer Detect. Prev*, 14(2):227–229.

Chapter IV

Prevention and Therapy of Liver Diseases

The economic burden of HBV infection is substantial because of the high morbidity and mortality associated with end stage liver disease, cirrhosis, and HCC. Costs escalate with increasing severity of illness. Because such serious liver problems develop over a number of years, direct medical costs as well as indirect costs attributable to lost work days and lost productivity are substantial.

HBV is not transmitted by hugging, kissing, sneezing or sharing eating or drinking utensils. It can be transmitted from infected people by: sharing intravenous drug paraphernalia; blood transfusion in countries that do not routinely screen donors; sexual intercourse without a condom; equipment from tattooing, body piercing or surgery including dentistry; sharing a toothbrush or shaving equipment.

Immunization with hepatitis B vaccine is the most effective means of preventing HBV infection and its consequences. It is quite possible that a course may give life-long immunity but for heath professionals a booster every 5 years is recommended in those with good antibody response. Antibody titres should be tested in health professionals 2 to 4 months after the primary course. Even with immunization it is essential to take all necessary precautions to prevent transmission of the virus. HBIG provides temporary protection (i.e., 3-6 months) and is indicated only in certain postexposure settings. HBIG is prepared from plasma known to contain a high titer of antibody against HBsAg (anti-HBs). In the United States, HBIG has an anti-HBs titer of >100,000 by radioimmunoassay. The human plasma from which HBIG is prepared is screened for antibodies to

HIV; in addition, the process used to prepare HBIG inactivates and eliminates HIV from the final product. There is no evidence that HIV can be transmitted by HBIG.

1. Role of Vaccination in Controlling HBV Infection

Hepatitis B viral infection is a preventable disease. Vaccination is the most effective tool in preventing the transmission of HBV infection.a safe and effective vaccine, which has been available for more than 20 years, is 95% effective in preventing the development of chronic infection. Broader vaccination programs are required including infants, children, health care workers and pregnant women. In 1991, the World Health Organization (WHO) recommended adding HBV vaccination to all national immunization programs. By May 2002, 154 countries had routine infant immunization with hepatitis B vaccine (WHO).

Two types of hepatitis B vaccine have been licensed. One was manufactured from the plasma of chronically infected persons. The currently available vaccines are produced by recombinant DNA technology. The recombinant vaccines are produced by using HBsAg synthesized by Saccharomyces cerevisiae (common bakers' yeast), into which a plasmid containing the gene for HBsAg has been inserted. Purified HBsAg is obtained by lysing the yeast cells and separating HBsAg from the yeast components by biochemical and biophysical techniques. Hepatitis B vaccines are packaged to contain 10-40 ug of HBsAg protein/mL after adsorption to aluminum hydroxide (0.5mg/mL); thimerosal (1:20,000 concentration) is added as a preservative.

Efficacy of Vaccines

Hepatitis vaccines have two purposes: to prevent the morbidity and occasional mortality associated with acute hepatitis virus infection and to reduce the occurrence of chronic liver disease and hepatocellular carcinoma. Two general types of hepatitis B vaccine have been used widely: heat-inactivated or chemically inactivated subviral particles derived from plasma collected from chronic carriers of HBsAg (plasma-derived vaccine) and HBsAg particles expressed from recombinant DNA in the yeast *Saccharomyces cerevisiae* (recombinant vaccine). Protective serum titers of anti-HBs (10 mIU per milliliter) develop in 95 to 99 percent of healthy infants, children, and young adults who receive a series of three intramuscular doses. However, the anti-HBs response is reduced in persons who are over 40 years of age or are otherwise immunocompromised. [1-6] The recommended dosages and immunization schedules vary according to age, and patients who are immunocompromised or receiving hemodialysis should be given larger doses.

Well-designed clinical trials have demonstrated the efficacy of both plasma-derived and recombinant vaccines, but it has been suggested that existing vaccines may not protect against rare HBV variants with mutations in the S protein. [7-9] Such variants have been found in high-risk infants who became infected despite the administration of vaccine and hepatitis B immune globulin soon after birth.

Despite optimal vaccination schedules, approximately 5 to 10% of healthy adults fail to make a high-level antibody response to HBV. A considerable body of evidence indicates that antibody responsiveness to HBV is under genetic control. [10] An increasing number of new and improved vaccines are being introduced. A combined hepatitis A and B vaccine was licensed in Europe in 1996 and Canada a year later. This vaccine has been proven safe and immunogenic when given as a 3 dose schedule in children, adolescents and adults [11, 12].

The long term protection afforded by immunization reflects the normally lengthy incubation period of hepatitis B, which permits previously immunized persons to mount protective anamnestic antibody responses on exposure to virus. Analysis of non-responders to HBV vaccine has shown that genetic factors are important in determining the likelihood of mounting an antibody response after vaccination. Meanwhile many conditions, such as HBV variants, alcoholism, chemotherapy, age, and HIV infection, etc., that affect the immune system are associated with significantly reduced antibody responses to the HBV vaccine.

It is very important to do postvaccination testing for serologic response. Postvaccination testing should be performed from 1 to 6 months after completion of the vaccine series. Although vaccination against hepatitis B virus (HBV) is highly successful, 5% to 10% of individuals do not experience a response with an adequate antibody level to hepatitis B surface antigen (anti-HBs) when persons who do not respond to the primary vaccine series are revaccinated, 15%-25% produce an adequate antibody response after one additional dose and 30%-50%

after three additional doses [13]. Therefore, revaccination with one or more additional doses should be considered for persons who do not respond to vaccination initially.

2. Treatment of HBV Infection

The need for treatment of hepatitis B depends on the natural history of the disease. Rates of progression to cirrhosis and hepatocellular carcinoma vary according to the state of the immune system, the age of the patient, the serologic stage of infection, and geographic and genetic factors. [14-17] There is little benefit in treating stage 1 infection with immunostimulants such as interferon, [18] nor is there a need to treat stage 3 or 4 infection. [19-21] The goal of treatment is to hasten the progression from stage 2 to stage 3, with the clearance of hepatocytes replicating virus, since they are the prime focus of the liver injury. [22] Spontaneous seroconversion occurs at a rate of approximately 5 percent per year. [23] It is interesting to note that seroconversion has occurred in patients receiving cells from a vaccinated person during bone marrow transplantation [24] and in HIV-positive patients with improved immunocompetence due to protease-inhibitor therapy. [25]

Histologic changes do not directly mirror the virologic stage of disease (figure 1a). For example, at stage 2, patients may have a variety of histologic features, from those of mild chronic hepatitis to those of advanced cirrhosis or hepatocellular carcinoma. At stages 1, 3, and 4, however, patients have minimal or no inflammation (figure 1b).

An anticipated effect of treatment is a further elevation of aminotransferase levels, occasionally to values of more than 1000 IU per liter, a response unlike that seen in hepatitis C (figure 2). About 10 percent of patients have a sustained disappearance of HBV DNA with the clearance of HBeAg later in the course of infection. The discordance between the responses of HBeAg and HBV DNA reflects the complexity of this process, as well as the use of more sensitive DNA assays. Persistently elevated enzyme levels despite HBeAg clearance suggests the presence of an HBeAg-negative mutant, which may emerge during treatment. This possibility requires confirmation with the measurement of HBV DNA levels.

Although chronic HBV infection is highly preventable through vaccination, once it has been established, the sole option for thwarting long-term liver disease is treatment.

2.1. IFNa

2.1.1. Conventional IFNa in the Treatment of Chronic Hepatitis B

In contrast to nucleoside and nucleotide analogues, conventional IFNa has a dual mode of action involving immunomodulatory actions as well as antiviral activity [26]. The immunomodulatory properties of conventional IFNa that can alter the course of chronic HBV infection include activation or induction of macrophages, natural killer cells, and cytotoxic T cells, and modulation of antibody production. Antiviral activity includes the induction of the enzyme 2,5-oligo adenyl synthetase and induction of protein kinase.

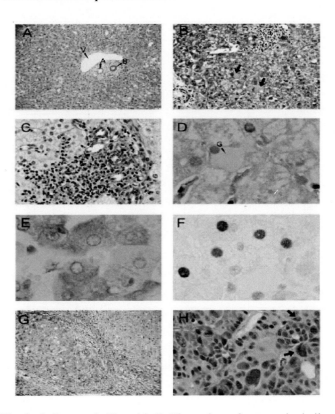

Figure 4.1. Histologic Patterns in Hepatitis B. The variety of patterns is similar to the spectrum of changes observed in other forms of chronic viral hepatitis. Panel A shows a section of normal liver with a portal triad containing a normalappearing bile duct (B), arteriole (A), and venule (V) (hematoxylin and eosin, 40 ×). Panel B shows the features of chronic hepatitis B with mild activity. Only rare piecemeal necrosis is seen, and no fibrosis

is present. The few lobular hepatocytes with ground-glass cytoplasm (arrows) are typical of virus-containing cells (Masson's trichrome, 100 ×). Panel C shows the features of chronic hepatitis B with moderate-to-severe activity. Piecemeal necrosis with spillover of the portal tract inflammatory cells into the lobule involves more than 50 percent of the portal tract perimeter (periodic acid–Schiff, 200×). Panel D shows a groundglass cell (G). The single cell in the center with homogeneous cytoplasm contains large quantities of HBsAg (hematoxylin and eosin, 1000 ×). Panel E shows specific immunoperoxidase staining (brown) for HBsAg, with cytoplasmic and a small amount of membranous HBsAg (avidin–biotin complex, 1000 ×). Panel F shows specific immunoperoxidase staining for HBcAg, with nucleocapsid staining confined to the hepatocyte nuclei (avidin–biotin complex, 1000 ×). Panel G shows cirrhosis due to chronic hepatitis B. Thick fibrous bands surround regenerative nodules, with mild chronic inflammation (Masson's trichrome, 200 ×). Panel H shows the features of moderately differentiated hepatocellular carcinoma. The tumor cells simulate liver cells and form small rosettes. Numerous mitotic figures (arrows) are present (hematoxylin and eosin, 600 ×).

2.1.2. Response to Treatment of HBeAg-Positive Chronic Hepatitis B with Conventional IFNa

Four to 6 months of therapy with conventional IFNa-2a (2.5, 5.0 and 10 MIU thrice weekly) has produced encouraging results, with rates of HBeAg loss of 20–50% [27-29]. Response to treatment with conventional IFNa is sustained, as approximately 90% of end-of-treatment responders maintain a positive response [28-30]. A study conducted at the National Institute of Health confirmed that a sustained response was maintained following treatment with conventional IFNa (patients were followed for a mean of 4.3 years). HBeAg loss was followed by loss of HBsAg in 87% of patients after conventional IFNa therapy [31]. Conventional IFNa has been shown to have beneficial long-term effects on disease outcome, incidence of HCC development and complication-free survival [32-35].

Interferon is a naturally occurring peptide that modulates immune function, often involved in the control or elimination of acute and chronic viral infections by the host. In addition to its immunomodulatory activity, interferon has broad antiviral properties. Several clinical trials have shown effectiveness of interferon in patients with CHB. In a meta-analysis of 15 randomized, placebo-controlled trials significantly more patients treated with IFN-a 2b achieved hepatitis B e antigen (HBeAg) loss (33% vs. 12%), reduction of HBV DNA level below the quantifiable limit by hybridization assay (37% *vs* 17%), and HBsAg loss (8% *vs* 2%). [36] Severalstudies in Asian [37,38] and predominantly Caucasian [39,40] populations have shown that interferon responders have a better prognosis than nonresponders, with a lower risk of progression of liver fibrosis, a higher rate of

HBsAg loss, and a higher rate of survival. In contrast, a study of HBeAg-positive Chinese patients by Yuen et al. [41] failed to show any benefit of interferon therapy in preventing longterm cirrhosis-related complications. In this study, however, a significant proportion of patients underwent HBeAg seroreversion with reemergence of HBV DNA, and HBeAg seroreversion rate was higher in the interferon-treated group compared with a control group (21.1% vs 2.2%) [41].

Similar conclusions can be drawn from studies of HBeAg-negative patients. Lampertico et al. [42] demonstrated a rate of sustained viral suppression (by dot-blot hybridization assay) and normalization of ALT levels in 33% of a cohort of HBeAg-negative patients treated with IFN-a 2b 6 MU TIW for 24 months (though earlier studies showed higher rates of relapse and, consequently, lower sustained response rates with shorter durations of therapy in these patients). Papatheodoridis et al. [43] showed improved clinical outcomes in HBeAg-negative patients successfully responding to interferon when compared to nonresponders.

Patients more likely to respond to interferon are those who have low serum HBV DNA, high serum ALT, high histologic activity, and more severe necroinflammation on liver biopsy independent of HBeAg status. Response rates may also vary according to HBV genotype, with recent evidence indicating superior efficacy in HBV genotypes A and B compared with C and D. [44] Proponents of interferon argue that it involves a finite course of therapy unassociated with the risk of selection for resistant mutations, and that its broad mechanisms of action may account for the loss of HBsAg in 5%–8% of interferon- treated patients, an outcome much less frequently seen after 1 year of oral antiviral therapy. Interferon is contraindicated in patients with decompensated cirrhosis because of the risk of a hepatitis flare leading to liver failure and should be used with caution even in compensated cirrhotics. [45]

2.1.3. Response to Treatment of HBeAg-Negative Chronic Hepatitis B with Conventional IFNa

Hepatitis B e antigen-negative CHB is less susceptible to therapy than HBeAg-positive 'wild-type' virus and is associated with a poorer prognosis. Therefore, treatment needs to be given early during the natural course of HB infection before mutation to the HBeAg-negative variant occurs, thereby preventing the HBeAg-negative variant from becoming the prevalent form of the virus. Severe disease progresses quickly with HBeAg-negative HBV; 60% of patients with this form of disease develop cirrhosis within 6 years [35].

After up to 12 months of therapy, approximately 50–70% of patients treated with conventional IFNa showed a positive response (normalization of ALT values and disappearance of HBV DNA). [35,46,47] However, data from various studies indicate that sustained response rates are highly variable, with 6–24% of patients maintaining a sustained response (12–18 months after cessation of therapy) [46, 47]. A longer duration of therapy has been shown to improve response rates. Indeed, in one study, an end-of-follow-up sustained response was achieved in 33% of patients who received 24 months of conventional IFNa therapy. [42] Long-term follow-up analyzes suggest that sustained response is maintained in a modest percentage of patients. In a Greek study of 209 patients, 27.3% of them maintained a sustained clinical response after a mean follow-up period of 6 years. [43] Results of a large retrospective analysis showed that 54% of the 216 patients who had received conventional IFNa for the first time had normal ALT levels and undetectable HBV DNAat the end of treatment. [46] Although 56%of initial responders relapsed after discontinuing conventional IFNa, 33% of initial responders were still in remission at the end of the follow-up period (median follow-up 7 years). HBeAg-negative CHB patients with a sustained response to therapy had a significantly improved disease outcome and complication-free survival compared with non-sustained responders. [43]

2.1.4. Influence of Conventional IFNa on the Natural History of Chronic Hepatitis B

Treatment with conventional IFNa not only results in loss of viremia and normalization of liver enzymes, but also improves long-term outcomes and survival, and alters the natural history of the disease. In addition, treatment with conventional IFNa was also associated with improved outcome of HBeAg-negative CHB (P < 0.001), reducing by 2.5-fold the risk of disease progression as assessed by cirrhosis or end-stage complications of cirrhosis. [35] Patients with HBeAg-positive CHB followed for up to 20 years, who achieved sustained virological and biochemical remission with IFNa therapy, also had a decreased incidence of liverrelated complications and improved 5-year survival, even when liver-compensated cirrhosis was present. [43] Furthermore, in patients with HBeAg-negative CHB, sustained biochemical remission resulting from IFNa treatment was associated with significantly improved overall and complication-free survival (P 0.027 and P0.019) [43].

2.1.5. Nucleoside and Nucleotide Analogues in the Treatment of Chronic Hepatitis B

Nucleoside/nucleotide analogues suppress HBV replication through inhibition of HBV DNA polymerase [26,48]. Nucleotide analogues inhibit HBV DNA replication through various combinations of interference with base priming, reverse transcription of the pregenomic messenger RNA to new minus strand DNA, or formation of new positive strand DNA from the minus strand DNA template. In most cases, they must be given for more than 1 year to achieve maximal efficacy. However, drug resistance can occur with prolonged therapy.

2.2. Lamivudine

Lamivudine 100 mg daily has good tolerability and an excellent safety profile. HBeAg seroconversion can be demonstrated in 16%–18% and HBeAg loss in 17%–33% of patients after 1 year of therapy.[49-52] Extending lamivudine therapy beyond 1 year increases rates of seroconversion; however, it has been associated with increasing lamivudine resistance due to emergence of lamivudine-resistant YMDD viral strains with mutation resulting in a methionine to valine or isoleucine substitution (rtM204V/I).[53,54] Four-year treatment data on 58 Chinese patients showed HBeAg seroconversion rate of 22%, 29%, 40%, and 47% at 1, 2, 3, and 4 years, respectively. However, the proportion of patients with YMDD mutation also increased with increasing duration of treatment from 17% after 1 year of treatment to 40%, 57%, and 67% after 2, 3, and 4 years of treatment, respectively. [55] Appearance of YMDD variants may be associated with increases in serum HBV DNA and ALT toward the pretreatment levels as well as reversal of initial histologic improvement. [54]

Current data suggest that discontinuation of lamivudine can be considered in patients who have sustained HBeAg seroconversion, completed at least 1 year of treatment and at least an additional 6 months of therapy after HBeAg seroconversion has been confirmed on repeat testing. Additional lamivudine therapy for >4 months after HBeAg seroconversion significantly decreased the relapse rate in Korean patients, [56] while Chien et al. suggest that even longer (>8 months) therapy may be required to ensure higher sustained response. [57] The same authors [57] suggested that patients with genotype B have a much higher sustained response than those with genotype C infection (61% vs 25%).

The potential for nucleoside analogues to improve long-term adverse clinical outcomes in CHB was demonstrated in a prospective randomized trial involving 651 HBeAg-positive and -negative predominantly Asian patients with advanced fibrosis or cirrhosis (liver biopsy showing an Ishak fibrosis score of at least 4) and detectable viral load (determined by a branchedchain hybridization assay with a lower limit of detection of 0.7 mEq per ml).[58] Lamivudine significantly reduced the rate of disease progression (8% vs 18%) and development of HCC (4% vs 7%) compared to placebo after a median of 32 months; however, 49% of patients developed lamivudine resistance, and clinical benefit was less apparent in this subset of patients. This landmark study demonstrated for the first time that persistent suppression of HBV halts disease progression in early cirrhosis. As with interferon, as well as other oral agents studied subsequently, patients with higher baseline serum ALT are more likely to undergo HBeAg seroconversion independent of ethnicity. [49-52] Unlike interferon, lamivudine is efficacious in chronic HBeAg-negative infection, with short-term therapy (24 weeks) achieving ALT/biochemical response rates similar to those in HBeAg-positive patients. [59] However most HBeAg-negative patients relapse shortly after treatment stopped, while continued therapy leads to the emergence of YMDD mutants associated with increasing serum HBV DNA level and ALT [60].

2.2.1. Response to Treatment of HBeAg-Positive Chronic Hepatitis B with Conventional with Lamivudine

After 12 months of therapy with lamivudine 100 mg daily, end-of-treatment seroconversion rates (disappearance of HBeAg and appearance of anti-HBe) range from 17 to 21% [49-51]. However, reversion to HBeAg-positive status after cessation of lamivudine therapy has been observed, and a positive response (sustained response 2 years after cessation of therapy) is maintained in 50% of end-of-treatment responders to lamivudine therapy [56].

2.2.2. Response to Treatment of HBeAg-negative Chronic Hepatitis B with Conventional with Lamivudine

Lamivudine shows moderate 1-year response rates in patients with HBeAg-negative CHB disease. Lamivudine demonstrates a positive response (ALT normalization and HBV DNA suppression) in 65–87% of patients after 12 months of therapy, and in 40% of patients at the end of 30 months of continuous treatmen [59-61]. However, in the majority of patients, a positive response is not maintained when treatment is stopped; only 13–17% of patients show a sustained response 6 months after cessation of therapy [59-62]. Lamivudine therapy produced favorable effects on histological features of HBV infection. In a 52-week, randomized, placebo-controlled US efficacy study of 143 patients, 52% of patients in the lamivudine group had a reduction of at least two points in the Histologic Activity Index (HAI) compared with 23% of those in the placebo group (P < 0.001) [50]. However, the clinical relevance of a two-point drop in the HAI score has not yet been defined.

2.3. Adefovir Dipivoxil

The adenine nucleotide analogue adefovir dipivoxil is an oral antiviral drug with activity against both wild-type and lamivudine-resistant HBV [63-65]. A 48-week course of treatment with adefovir (10 mg daily for chronic therapy) in patients with HBeAg-positive CHB resulted in significant reductions in HBV DNA levels. However, the HBeAg seroconversion rate was only 12% at 48 weeks, increasing to 21% when treatment was continued to 100 weeks. At this time, HBV DNA was undetectable and ALT levels had normalized in 70% of patients. In a separate multicentre study, adefovir treatment was associated with significant histological improvement, but again, the HBeAg seroconversion rate was only 12% at 48 weeks [66]. Adefovir was found to have similar antiviral efficacy against all types of HBV, including lamivudine-resistant YMDD mutant HBV strains [64, 67, 68], but a recent study has demonstrated low level resistance to adefovir treatment after 96 weeks of therapy. Similar to lamivudine, patients experience a viral rebound on cessation of therapy. There is no evidence that sustained responses and HBsAg clearance can be achieved with adefovir monotherapy. Although a promising drug, further studies will have to determine the long-term efficacy of adefovir and its potential to be combined with other drugs.

Adefovir dipivoxil is the first nucleotide analogue approved for treatment (in 2002) of HBeAg-positive and HBeAg-negative CHB. In the registration trial of adefovir 10 mg daily in HBeAg-positive patients, HBeAg seroconversion and HBeAg loss occurred in 12% and 24%, respectively. [66] Cumulative incidence of adefovir resistance was much more favorable with 0% at 48 weeks and only 2% at 2 years. [69] The two predominant mutations in the HBV DNA polymerase associated with adefovir resistance are N236T and A181T. Among HBeAg-negative patients, after 48 weeks of therapy HBV DNA was undetectable in 51% [70] and reached 71% with continued therapy at 96 weeks. [71] As with lamivudine, the pivotal trials with adefovir therapy for 1 year demonstrated significant histologic benefit compared with placebo.

Addition of adefovir to ongoing lamivudine therapy, or replacement of lamivudine with adefovir, was shown to be effective in suppressing lamivudine-resistant HBV [72, 73] in several clinical trials. Although there was no difference in virologic, or biochemical response among those who received adefovir alone compared to those who received adefovir in addition to lamivudine, patients who received adefovir alone had more flares in ALT compared to the combination therapy group. Because of these findings, a 1–3 month overlap period became a commonly advised practice, especially in patients with cirrhosis.

2.4. Entecavir

The guanosine nucleoside analogue entecavir is an oral antiviral drug with activity against both wild-type and lamivudine-resistant HBV. [74,75] In a 28-day, randomized, placebo-controlled, dose-escalating, phase 1/2 study, a pronounced decrease of HBV DNA was observed and there were no significant side-effects. [74] The drug is currently being evaluated in phase 3 clinical trials.

2.5. Pegylated IFNa

Pegylated IFNa was developed through the process of pegylation, in which a polyethylene glycol (PEG) polymer molecule is attached to the base IFNa molecule to produce a drug with a prolonged half-life. In the last few years, there have been extensive trials carried out with two larger polymers, namely, the 12 kDa PEG, with linkage of IFNa-2b to a linear PEG molecule, and the 40 kDa branched PEG linked to IFNa-2a. The binding sites of the two molecules differ, and thus the stability of these molecules also differ both in vitro and in vivo. Furthermore, the different size of the two molecules leads to different volumes of distribution, the organs in which the drug is distributed, and its sites of catabolism. In short, the peginterferon alfa-2a (40 kDa) (PEG IFNa-2a) has a longer half-life (>100 h), and its breakdown products are biologically active. It is largely restricted to the liver where it is metabolized. Peginterferon alfa-2b (12 kDa) (PEG IFNa-2b) has a shorter half-life and is somewhat more of a prodrug acting as a depot of IFNa with the release of free IFNa. [76] Peginterferon alfa-2b (12 kDa) is widely distributed. The two pegylated IFNs have been used in a variety of trials in patients with chronic hepatitis C, and results show considerable improvement in efficacy over conventional IFNa [77-80] raising the question as to whether pegylated IFNs would be of use in patients with CHB. Data for PEG IFNa-2a (40 kDa) are now available on patients with CHB. Preliminary results indicate that more than twice as many HBeAgpositive patients receiving PEG IFNa-2a (40 kDa) 180 lg weekly for 6 months achieved the combined response (HBeAg loss, HBV DNA <500 000 copies/mL, ALT normalization) compared with patients receiving conventional IFNa-2a, (28 and 12%, respectively). [81] Patients treated with PEG IFNa-2a (40 kDa) for 6 months had substantially higher rates of HBeAg clearance and seroconversion than did patients treated with conventional IFNa-2a (33% *vs* 25%). Of particular interest is the finding of improved responses to PEG IFNa-2a (40 kDa) in those patients traditionally considered to have difficult-to-treat HBV infection, such as those with low pretreatment ALT levels and high pretreatment HBV DNA levels. Within this group of patients response rates were also substantially higher in those patients treated with PEG IFNa-2a (40 kDa) than in those treated with conventional IFNa-2a (figure 4). Validation of these promising results is eagerly awaited from ongoing, large-scale, multicentre trials in both HBeAg positive and HBeAg-negative patients. In addition, these studies will hopefully clarify whether the combination of lamivudine and PEG IFNa-2a (40 kDa) is better than monotherapy with PEG IFNa-2a (40 kDa) in the treatment of CHB.

2.6. Potential of Combination Therapy

2.6.1. Lamivudine and IFNa Combination Therapy

Lamivudine in combination with conventional IFNa appears to be more effective than either agent alone in increasing the rate of HBeAg seroconversion. In a comparison of the three treatments in patients with HBeAg-positive chronic HBV infection, the HBeAg seroconversion rates after 52 weeks of therapy were 29% for combination therapy, 18% for lamivudine monotherapy, and 19% for conventional IFNa-2a monotherapy. [51] Clinical trials of combination therapy with PEG IFNa-2a (40 kDa) are currently under way and the results are eagerly awaited.

2.6.2. Peginterferon Alfa, Lamivudine, or Combination Therapy

In a multicenter, partially double-blind study by Lau et al.[44] conducted at 67 sites in 16 countries in Asia, Australia, Europe, and North and South America, patients were randomized to peginterferon alfa-2a (180 mcg) once weekly plus oral placebo once daily, peginterferon once weekly plus lamivudine (100 mg) once daily, or lamivudine once daily for 48 weeks. Most patients were Asian (87%) and were predominantly infected with genotype B or C. After 24 weeks of follow-up, HBeAg seroconversion rate was significantly higher among patients who received peginterferon alfa-2a monotherapy or peginterferon alfa-2a with lamivudine than those who received lamivudine monotherapy (32% vs 19% and 27% vs 19%, respectively), as was the number of patients with HBV DNA < 100,000 copies/ml (32% vs 22% and 34% vs 22% , respectively). Response rates varied with HBV genotype, with superior efficacy in HBV genotypes A and B compared with C and D. At week 72, HBsAg seroconversion occurred in 16 patients (2% of Asian and 17% of white patients) receiving peginterferon with, or without lamivudine, and in 0% receiving lamivudine alone. The rate of histologic response at 72 weeks was similar in the 3 treatment groups, although it did correlate closely with HBeAg seroconversion (74% vs 41%). Interestingly, rates of YMDD mutation were significantly lower in the combination compared to lamivudine monotherapy group (27% vs 4%) after 48 weeks. The most common adverse events were those known to be related to interferon-alfa therapy; however, incidence of depression was significantly lower than that reported in hepatitis C trials (5% vs 16%–20%). [77, 82] Although peginterferon seems to be more effective than lamivudine monotherapy, rate of viral response decreases with time such that 25%–69% of peginterferon-treated patients have HBV DNA < 400 copies/ml at the end of treatment (week 48), compared to 14% at the end of follow-up at week 72. [44] Longer follow-up data is needed to define a true efficacy of peginterferon in the management of chronic hepatitis B.

The suppressive anti-viral therapy improves the natural history of HBV [83-85]. Interferon therapy remains sustained remission rates remain relatively low, so some researches are undergoing to identify the host single nucleotide polymorphisms (SNPs) that predict IFN response in hepatitis B patients or the relationship between IFN gene polymorphism and susceptibility to HBV infection [86,87].

SNPs, on the other hand, are stable, common and increasingly amenable to high throughput automated genotyping. A number of studies have sought genetic associations between HBV infection/persistence and gene polymorphisms (Tables 1 and 2). The prototype region for genetic association studies is the human leukocyte antigen (HLA) loci involved in antigen processing and presentation. This is most obvious within the HLA region, where functional variation has arisen as a strategy to combat pathogen antigenic diversity. Indeed in HBV infection, maximal HLA variation appears to have a direct protective effect, individuals with the most different alleles at class II HLA loci have the slowest HBV disease progression and the lowest mortality (a "heterozygous advantage"). [88] Conversely, lack of HLA diversity (a "homozygous disadvantage") may increase the susceptibility to HBV infection among isolated communities. [89] The extensive linkage disequilibrium across some HLA regions makes it difficult to localize specific disease-associated polymorphisms, although the HLA allelic association has allowed identifi cation of criticall pathogenic epitopes in some diseases, [90] which might act as potential vaccine candidates. The goal of therapy in chronic HBV infection is to eliminate or significantly suppress HBV replication and prevent the progression of liver disease to cirrhosis with the potential development of liver failure or HCC [91].

In recent years many people focused on the development and manufacture of DNA-based vaccines for HBV. Due to the induction of strong CTL, DNA vaccines may be effective for the treatment of chronic carriers of HBV. Some HBV DNA vaccines have been used in the preliminary clinical trials and exhibited exciting results in chronic HBV carriers. Some vaccines encoded the viral antigen, the S or the PreS2/S antigen, hepatitis B core antigen, or both antigens. Patients with chronic hepatitis B show a state of relative hypo-responsiveness of HBV-specific T cells compared with that demonstrated in patients who control the virus replication after acute infection. Therapeutic induction and/or activation of the T-cell response for HBV core and surface proteins may have the potential to control infection. It has been shown that Hepatitis B surface (HBsAg) and core antigen (HBcAg) induces envelope-and core specific CD4+ and CD8+ T-cell responses and that the response against the Hepatitis B core antigen (HBcAg), is often associated with viral control. The combination of these two genes in PowderMed's pdpSC18 HBV therapeutic DNA vaccine, thus provides a potential mechanism to both clear the virus via the CD8+ response and to overcome unresponsiveness in chronically infected patients via the CD4+ response.

3. Recurrent Hepatitis B after Liver Transplantation

3.1. Recurrent Hepatitis B

Hepatitis B-related liver disease is a major cause of end-stage liver disease, for which liver transplantation is the only treatment option. However, the success of liver transplantation is limited by the high incidence of recurrent graft infection and subsequent graft failure, and rapid progression to cirrhosis and fibrosing cholestatic hepatitis or fulminant hepatitis.

The use of nucleoside analogs has been shown to prevent liver failure as well as prolonging transplant free survival in patients with chronic hepatitis. [92-96] However, if cirrhosis and liver failure develops, the definitive treatment of choice remains orthotopic liver transplantation (OLT). An unacceptable recurrence rate with an extremely high rate of graft loss was noted initially and HBV infection was actually considered to be a relative contraindication to OLT. [97-99] Fortunately, the use of HBIG resulted in markedly improved patient and graft survival rates. The addition of the nucleoside analog Lamivudine (LAM) to Hepatitis B Immunoglobulin (HBIG) has improved these survival curves to an even greater degree (greater than 80% five year survival rate) while also enabling the treatment team to consider discontinuation of the costly HBIG preparation.[100]

In the pre-transplant setting prolonged use of LAM will almost invariably lead to the development of viral mutations resistant to the drug. Furthermore, prolonged therapy with LAM in the post-transplant setting could also lead to the development of LAM-resistant mutants. Indeed, there have now been several reports of these mutations developing following OLT. [101-110] This raises the question of how to treat these LAM-resistant patients in the post-transplant period. Fortunately, there are other nucleoside and nucleotide analogs (Adefovir, Entecavir, Tenofovir, and Truvada) available now or in the near future for the clinician.

Several studies showed that the following factors influence the HBV recurrence after OLT [111-116]: the HBV infection before surgery, the administration of immunosuppressive agents, the HBV level in extrahepatic tissues and the genotype of HBV. It is generally accepted that patients with active replication of HBV before the surgery and on high dose immunosuppressive agents are easier to be reinfected.

3.2. Prevention of HBV Recurrence

3.2.1. Hepatitis B Immunoglobulin (HBIG)

HBIG first became available for use in 1975. This agent provides a means of passive immunity for the patient. In principle, polyvalent anti-HBs antibodies will bind to and neutralize circulating virions and prevent subsequent graft infection. Anti-HBs also undergoes endocytosis by hepatocytes and binds to HBsAg within cells already infected, thereby decreasing HBsAg secretion. The first large study demonstrating the efficacy of long term HBIG came from the EUROHEP study group in 1993. Three hundred seventy-two patients transplanted for HBV-related liver failure were observed. The risk of HBV recurrence was 75 ± 6% among the 67 patients given no immunoprophylaxis, 74 ± 5 percent among the 83 treated for two months, and 36 ± 4 percent among the 209 treated for six months or longer (P < 0.001). Improved patient survival (75 versus 45 percent) at three years was also noted among those patients receiving passive prophylaxis with HBIG. Multivariate analysis revealed that long-term administration of HBIG was associated with a relative risk reduction of 3.3 for the development of recurrent HBV. [111] These findings have now been confirmed in multiple studies and the median rate of recurrent HBV in patients receiving longterm HBIG is approximately 20% over one to two years. [117-126]

There are several drawbacks to the use of HBIG. First is its cost. Most regimens currently in use in the United States range from $80,000 to $200,000 for the first year. These costs also include the cumbersome IV infusion sets and monitoring of the patient during administration. [122] The supply of HBIG is limited. Significant side effects have been noted with the infusion including headaches, flushing and chest pain. [117].Lastly, the development of escape mutants can be seen reducing the efficacy of HBIG. These escape mutants are typically due to mutation in the HBsAg at the "a" determinant loop. [127]The trend has been toward lower doses given intramuscularly.

In the past, the use of monoclonal antibody to the HBV surface antigen led to an unacceptable rate of breakthrough infections. [128] However, a recent study by Galun et.al [129] showed promising results using a mixture of two monoclonal antibodies in a phase I clinical study. Patients developed a rapid and significant decrease in HBV-DNA levels. Future studies are warranted, but this preliminary data suggests that monoclonal antibody preparations could replace the current polyclonal HBIG.

Intravenous hepatitis B immune globulin (HBIg) is the first agent to reduce the recurrence of hepatitis B virus (HBV) and improve graft survival after liver transplantation. The landmark study by Samuel [111] revealed that HBV infection could be reduced in frequency when a high dose of HBIg was used for more than 6 months after liver transplantation. The beneficial effect of HBIg is more likely to be achieved in the patients who lack evidence for viral replication. Some obstacles to acceptance of long-term HBIg also include side-effects, expensive treatment, uncertain dose of the agent, and duration of the treatment. Most of HBIg failures are due to the selection pressure on the surface antigen gene, leading to the development of mutants. [130-131] HBIg monotherapy against HBV recurrence for active viral replication, about half allografts will lose their function within 3 years. [111]

3.2.2. Lamivudine (LAM)

Lamivudine (LAM) was the first nucleoside analog to be approved for the use of chronic HBV. Its mechanism of action is the inhibition of the DNA polymerase of the virus and suppression of HBV replication. [49,132] LAM has also been shown to be safe in patients with decompensated liver disease; it is well tolerated and achieves a rapid loss of HBV DNA in the serum. LAM is preferred over the use of the Interferons which are contraindicated in patients with advanced cirrhosis. [92-96].

In the pre-transplant setting, the drug has been shown to be potent. Undetectable HBV DNA can be achieved in most patients within 2–3 months. [92,95, 96,101,133-140]. Furthermore, histologic improvement may be seen in 49–56% of patients after receiving one year of therapy.[50,51,127,141,142] Yao showed that the use of LAM could also improve the Child-Pugh-Turcotte (CPT) score by more than or equal to three points in 60% of patients receiving the drug and even reduce the necessity for OLTx. [96]

The major drawback to the use of LAM is the development of resistance to the drug caused by mutations in the reverse transcriptase gene. The most common mutations occur in Domain C of the HBV polymerase at the tyrosinemethionine-aspartate-aspartate (YMDD) locus. Other mutations can occur at Domain B in conjunction with the YMDD mutations. [143] Liaw showed that the cumulative rates of LAM resistance were 14%, 38%, 49%, 66% and 69%, one, two, three, four, and five years after initial therapy respectively. [144]Other studies have showed similar rates of resistance with resistance rates of 24% and 70% after one and four years of therapy respectively. [141,142,145]

In an attempt to lower the cost, and avoid the side effects and cumbersome administration of HBIG, multiple studies have examined the use of LAM prior to and following transplant to prevent HBV recurrence. Perillo *et al.* conducted the largest multicenter study in North America in which 77 liver transplant candidates were treated with LAM (100 mg daily) without the adjunctive use of HBIG. Treatment was initiated prior to and after transplantation. Forty-seven eventually underwent liver transplantation. Re-infection with HBV occurred at a rate of 40% over the subsequent three years and HBV-DNA polymerase mutants were detected in 15 (21%) of the transplanted patients. [95] Other studies with LAM monotherapy have also been disappointing with high rates of HBV recurrence ranging from 23–50% of patients.[134,136,146-148] The high rates of recurrence were due to the expected emergence of escape mutations in the YMDD locus. For this reason, LAM prophylactic monotherapy has been abandoned in favor of combination therapy with HBIG.

Lamivudine is a nucleoside analog that causes chain termination of HBV-DNA polymerase and inhibits viral reverse transcriptase. In immunosuppressed patients lamivudine has demonstrated its safety and efficacy in reducing HBV replication.[95,101,137,149] But with the development of lamivudine-resistant mutations in the YMDD region of the HBV-DNA polymerase, the recurrence rate of HBV has been increased by more than 25%.[efficacy in reducing HBV replication.[95,101,137,149] But with the development of lamivudine-resistant mutations in the YMDD region of the HBV-DNA polymerase, the recurrence rate of HBV has been increased by more than 25%.[150]

3.2.3. Lamivudine and Hepatitis B Immunoglobulin Combination Therapy

In contrast to monotherapy, LAM in combination with HBIG has been potent in preventing the recurrence of HBV in the post-transplant setting. Indeed, following the results of several studies, the standard of care has become administration of LAM in the pre-transplant setting (ideally, at least four weeks prior to transplantation) followed by the combination of LAM and HBIG in the post-transplant setting. HBV recurrence rates are usually less than 10% one to two years following transplantation. Furthermore, HBV DNA levels by PCR are also typically undetectable. [101, 133,135, 137,151-155]

These favorable response rates are likely secondary to the additive effects of LAM with the HBIG. Another added benefit of combination therapy is that HBIG can be administered in reduced amounts thus reducing costs and increasing availability of HBIG .[101,133] Some have argued that HBIG could even be stopped at some point after transplantation. This issue represents an impending controversy that requires further investigation before a robust recommendation can be made, although our center often discontinues HBIG at some point following OLT depending upon the individual patient, serologic studies and viral load.

3.2.4. Adefovir (ADV)

It is now well known that a significant number of patients can develop LAM resistant strains of HBV while receiving this drug in the pre-transplant setting. Furthermore, an increasing number of patients may become primarily infected with a LAM resistant HBV mutant. In this setting, the use of LAM for prevention of recurrent HBV in the post transplant setting is of limited value. Adefovir dipivoxil (ADV) is an orally available prodrug of Adefovir- a nucleotide analog of adenosine monophosphate that has been shown to have activity against both wild type and LAM resistant HBV.Improvement in histology, LFT's and viral DNA levels have been seen with the use of this drug. [66,156,157].The drug is very well tolerated and the only significant side effect is risk of increased nephrotoxicity after 20 or more weeks of use. [158]

Several large studies have shown the utility of ADV in the pre and post liver transplantation setting. The largest study by Schiff et al. showed that among patients with LAM-resistant HBV and who were pre-OLT, 81% achieved undetectable serum HBV DNA. Furthermore, serum ALT, Albumin, bilirubin and prothrombin time normalized in 76%, 81%, 50% and 83% of these pre-OLT patients respectively. Furthermore, the Child-Pugh-Turcotte score improved in over 90% of cohorts. Unlike the use of LAM, no resistance to ADV was identified after 48 weeks of therapy in this population.[159] Many patients came off the transplant list because of reversal of the decompensated state.

Another study describing the use of prophylactic ADV was from Lo et. al. They describe 16 patients who had developed YMDD mutations while on the waiting list for OLT. Eleven patients received ADV for a median of 20 days (range 8–271 days) before transplantation while 5 patients started the drug at the time of OLT. The median follow-up period after OLT was 21.1 months (range 4.4–68.9 months). One patient died of a cause unrelated to HBV 12.2 months after transplantation. Fifteen patients (94%) were alive with the original graft. Pre-OLT HBV DNA levels at the time of breakthrough were available in 15 patients ranging from $2 \times 103 - 4.69 \times 109$ copies/mL (median 1.42×107). Lo's cohort was divided in half: eight patients received HBIG (in addition to ADV and LAM) for a median of 24 months whereas the other 8 patients received prophylaxis with ADV and LAM alone. All 16 patients cleared the HBV DNA and had no evidence of recurrence; furthermore, all remained HBeAg negative. The graft survival was 94% at a median follow up of 21 months. Lo concludes that add-on ADV plus LAM should be the "preferred approach in those patients who have already developed resistance to lamivudine so as to avoid the emergence of multiresistant viral strains." [160]

Previous studies reported a low rate of ADV resistanceoccurring in less than 2% of patients after 96 weeks. [63,152,161] However, the emergence of ADV resistant HBV mutants is now considered to be clinically significant over time when given as monotherapy; resistance has been reported in 18% of patients after 4 years of therapy and 22% after 2 years of therapy [162,163].

It is expected that the development of ADV mutations will similarly become a problem in the post-transplant setting. Villenueve recently reported the first case of a patient who developed sequential selection of LAM and ADV resistant strains of HBV in a liver transplantation patient. [108] The patient was a 52 year old Cambodian who was initially HBV DNA negative and HBsAg positive. He was given prophylactic HBIG alone in the peritransplant setting without any nucleoside analogs. Virologic breakthrough with LAM resistance mutations in L180M and M204V followed 20 months later. ADV was added to LAM and after reduction in DNA levels, LAM was discontinued and ADV was continued alone. A subsequent reversion to wild type took place. A second virologic breakthrough occurred after nearly two years of ADV monotherapy with the selection of the resistance mutation N236T of the D domain of the HBV polymerase. [108] Xiong et al. had recently described this mutation in 2/124 patients receiving chronic ADV therapy for two years. [63] LAM was reintroduced with ADV after which the patient developed undetectable levels of the virus.

Both the Schiff and Lo study suggest that ADV provides safe and effective prophylaxis in those patients with LAM resistant HBV infection.An area for future investigation is whether the use of ADV in combination with LAM should be utilized. There are several potential benefits with combination therapy. The chance for breakthrough mutations to either LAM or ADV is significantly less when the agents are used in combination. [160,163] Snow et.al observed a patient population of 467 patients with LAM-resistant HBV. He reported that resistance to ADV was only seen in those who stopped LAM. Fung et al. studied all HBV patients in a tertiary care center receiving ADV. He found that none of the patients receiving combination therapy (LAM + ADV) developed ADV resistance; among those who had switched to ADV monotherapy after combination therapy,5 of 18 patients (28%) developed resistance. [163]

Another potential benefit of combination therapy would be to eliminate the need for HBIG with its economic cost and potential toxic side effects (see discussion above). Note that in Lo's study, all eight patients who did not receive HBIG remained alive with normal chemistries at a median follow up of 15.1 months (range 4.4– 26). Furthermore, there was no histologic evidence of recurrence. Six of these eight had spontaneous HBsAg seroconversion. Although, two of the eight remained HBsAg positive, both had undetectable DNA levels with normal LFT's. The possibility of a viral breakthrough with resistance to both LAM and ADV should be low given the relatively low frequency of ADV resistance and lack of cross-resistance to LAM when given in combination. [160]The duration of HBIG therapy remains a contentious issue; to suggest its elimination altogether is controversial and worthy of further investigation.

3.3. Treatment of HBV Recurrence

3.3.1. Lamivudine

Prior to combination HBIG/LAM, graft infection was frequently seen. As described above, this was due to the high recurrence rates in patients who received HBIG or LAM as monotherapy alone or in those who received no prophylaxis at all. De Novo HBV is also seen in the post transplant setting. Fortunately, LAM is very effective in treating HBV infection of the graft and remains the first line agent. Perillo performed a large multicenter center of 52 HBVDNA positive patients. After one year of treatment, LAM resulted in a 68% loss of HBV serum DNA with an 11% HBeAg seroconversion. [164] Other studies have shown similar improvements with HBV-DNA negativity ranging from 75 to 100%, although HBeAg serum conversion is generally less than 30%. [165,166] This low rate of serum conversion is consistent with prior reports in the nontransplanted population. [66]

Unfortunately, breakthrough is seen just as in the nontransplanted population in up to 50% of patients within the first one to two years following transplantation [164-166]. It should be expected that with even longer follow up the development of LAM resistant mutants should approach 70%. Continuation of LAM for graft infection that develops while receiving prophylaxis with LAM ± HBIG is not indicated. Furthermore, the use of LAM as a primary treatment agent is ineffective for de novo graft infection with a LAM resistant mutant. In these scenarios, ADV should be initiated, although Tenofovir or Truvada may ultimately replace ADV pending future studies.

3.3.2. Adefovir

The beneficial effects of ADV in the chronic HBV population suggested that ADV may be helpful for the development of LAM-resistant mutants in the transplanted population receiving prophylactic combination therapy or in the development of de novo LAM-resistant HBV infection. Schiff *et.al* performed a large multicenter study investigating the utility of Adefovir examined two cohorts with LAM-resistant HBV infection. The beneficial results seen in the pre-OLT cohort described above were also found in the post-OLT population.

One hundred ninety-six patients were followed for a median of 56.1 weeks. After 24 and 48 weeks of therapy with ADV, a 3.1 and 3.4 drop in log PCR DNA levels was seen. In addition, 34% achieved undetectable serum HBV DNA levels. Serum ALT, albumin, bilirubin and prothrombin time normalized in 49%, 76%, 75% and 20% of these patients respectively. A 93% one year survival was seen. [159] Several studies and case reports have confirmed the efficacy of ADV in the setting LAM-resistant graft infection whether it be the development of a mutant while on prophylactic therapy or de novo LAM-resistant HBV graft infection. Multiple studies have shown that there is a low rate of HBeAg seroconversion when Adefovir is used for patients with chronic Hepatitis B. [151] This observation is also found in the post transplant infected patients.

ADV is thus both an effective and safe drug to treat graft infection and prevent clinical deterioration of patients affected with the development LAM resistant HBV graft denovo infection or for LAM-resistant breakthrough mutants. Neff's study [107] described a total of 14 patients who had the development of LAM resistant mutants. Nine patients were switched from LAM to ADV. The other 5 patients were treated with Tenofovir. Of the patients given ADV, one died during follow-up. Of the 8 alive, all but one had reductions in HBV DNA.Toniutto's study [110] describes one patient who developed de novo HBV graft infection. 3 months after treatment of LAM, LAM resistance developed. The patient was given two months of ADV plus LAM with HBsAg seroconversion and undetectable HBV DNA levels. Therapy was stopped thereafter and the patient remains HBV negative 13 months later.

None of these studies and case reports described any significant nephrotoxicity with the use of ADV. In post-OLT patients, there are multiple factors, in particular the use of calcineurin inhibitors, that contribute to renal dysfunction. Some patients did develop a rise in serum creatinine which was easily treated with reduced frequency dosing of ADV.

3.3.3. Entecavir and Tenofovir

Although ADV is generally well tolerated, there does exist a risk of nephrotoxicity with this agent. Furthermore, as described above, there exists the possibility of N263T and other ADV resistant mutants. In these cases, it may be desirable to use either Tenofovir Disoproxil Fumarate or Entecavir.

Entecavir is a carboxylic analogue of guanosine and is the most recently FDA approved drug for the treatment of chronic Hepatitis B. Like Adefovir, it has been shown to be a potent antiviral agent for the wild type and LAM-resistant forms of chronic HBV. [74,167,168] It is expected that Entecavir will be efficacious in the prevention and treatment of recurrent HBV following liver transplantation. The first reports of Entecavir's use in this setting are now being reported.

Tenofovir is currently only approved for use in HIV positive patients but has been to be effective for LAM resistant mutants and for those patients who have failed prior ADV and LAM. It is a nucleotide analogue and acts as a reverse transcriptase inhibitor. [169-171] Several case reports have now been reported in which Tenofovir produced a well tolerated, successful antiviral response in patients before and after OLT.

Taltavull describe a 54 year old male who developed YMDD mutations while receiving LAM therapy. ADV produced a suboptimal response: DNA levels were still positive after 8 months of therapy. His clinical status continued to decline with spontaneous bacterial peritonitis and worsening of CPT status. Tenofovir was then added and produced a rapid dramatic decline in DNA levels to undetectable levels 4 weeks after treatment. He continued on this treatment up to OLT after which time he received only HBIG, LAM and ADV. [172] The patient's outcome remained excellent 21 months following OLT.

In 2004, Neff et.al [109] reported the successful use of Tenofovir in patients who developed the Lam resistance following OLT. From June, 1998 through December, 2003, 25 patients transplanted for HBV were managed on chronic LAM therapy. Sixteen patients (64%) developed resistance to LAM between 10–85 months (median 26) following OLT. Eight of these patients were administered Tenofovir at a dose of 300 mg/day 1–66 months after the development of resistance. Therapy was continued for 14–26 (median 19.3) months. All 8 patients experienced DNA suppression with 7 having undetectable viral loads. Creatinine clearance was not impaired nor was any other adverse event reported. Both the Taltavull and Neff study suggest that Tenofovir is a safe and effective therapy for those patients who develop LAM-resistant mutants after OLT. It also stands to reason that the use of Truvada (Emtricitabine and Tenofovir) will also be useful in this setting; although, like Tenofovir, it is not yet FDA approved for this use.

References

[1]   Clements ML, Miskovsky E, Davidson M, Cupps T, Kumwenda N, Sandman LA, West D, Hesley T, Ioli V, Miller W, et al.(1994).Effect of age on the immunogenicity of yeast recombinant hepatitis B vaccines containing surface antigen (S) or PreS2 + S antigens. *J. Infect. Dis,* 170(3):510-516.

[2]   Wood RC, MacDonald KL, White KE, Hedberg CW, Hanson M, Osterholm MT. (1993).Risk factors for lack of detectable antibody following hepatitis B vaccination of Minnesota health care workers. *Jama,* 270(24):2935-2939.

[3]   Collier AC, Corey L, Murphy VL, Handsfield HH.(1988).Antibody to human immunodeficiency virus (HIV) and suboptimal response to hepatitis B vaccination. *Ann. Intern. Med,* 109(2):101-105.

[4]   Weber DJ, Rutala WA, Samsa GP, Santimaw JE, Lemon SM.(1985).Obesity as a predictor of poor antibody response to hepatitis B plasma vaccine. *Jama,* 254(22):3187-3189.

[5]   Shaw FE, Jr., Guess HA, Roets JM, Mohr FE, Coleman PJ, Mandel EJ, Roehm RR, Jr., Talley WS, Hadler SC. (1989).Effect of anatomic injection site, age and smoking on the immune response to hepatitis B vaccination. *Vaccine,* 7(5):425-430.

[6]   Winter AP, Follett EA, McIntyre J, Stewart J, Symington IS.(1994). Influence of smoking on immunological responses to hepatitis B vaccine. *Vaccine,* 12(9):771-772.

[7]   Waters JA, Kennedy M, Voet P, Hauser P, Petre J, Carman W, Thomas HC.(1992).Loss of the common "A" determinant of hepatitis B surface antigen by a vaccine-induced escape mutant. *J. Clin. Invest,* 90(6):2543-2547.

[8]   Carman WF, Zanetti AR, Karayiannis P, Waters J, Manzillo G, Tanzi E, Zuckerman AJ, Thomas HC.(1990).Vaccine-induced escape mutant of hepatitis B virus. *Lancet,* 336(8711):325-329.

[9]   Fortuin M, Karthigesu V, Allison L, Howard C, Hoare S, Mendy M, Whittle HC. (1994).Breakthrough infections and identification of a viral variant in Gambian children immunized with hepatitis B vaccine. *J. Infect. Dis,* 169(6):1374-1376.

[10] Pirofski LA, Casadevall A. (1998).Use of licensed vaccines for active immunization of the immunocompromised host. *Clin. Microbiol. Rev*, 11(1):1-26.

[11] Diaz-Mitoma F, Law B, Parsons J. (1999).A combined vaccine against hepatitis A and B in children and adolescents. *Pediatr. Infect. Dis. J*, 18(2):109-114.

[12] Thoelen S, Van Damme P, Leentvaar-Kuypers A, Leroux-Roels G, Bruguera M, Frei PC, Bakasenas V, Safary A. (1999). The first combined vaccine against hepatitis A and B: an overview. *Vaccine*,17(13-14):1657-1662.

[13] Hadler SC, Francis DP, Maynard JE, Thompson SE, Judson FN, Echenberg DF, Ostrow DG, O'Malley PM, Penley KA, Altman NL, et al. (1986).Long-term immunogenicity and efficacy of hepatitis B vaccine in homosexual men. *N. Engl. J. Med*, 315(4):209-214.

[14] Lok AS, Lai CL. (1988).A longitudinal follow-up of asymptomatic hepatitis B surface antigen-positive Chinese children. *Hepatology*, 8(5):1130-1133.

[15] Fattovich G, Giustina G, Schalm SW, Hadziyannis S, Sanchez-Tapias J, Almasio P, Christensen E, Krogsgaard K, Degos F, Carneiro de Moura M, et al. (1995).Occurrence of hepatocellular carcinoma and decompensation in western European patients with cirrhosis type B.The EUROHEP Study Group on Hepatitis B Virus and Cirrhosis. *Hepatology*, 21(1):77-82.

[16] Liaw YF, Tai DI, Chu CM, Chen TJ.(1988).The development of cirrhosis in patients with chronic type B hepatitis: a prospective study. *Hepatology*, 8(3):493-496.

[17] Villeneuve JP, Desrochers M, Infante-Rivard C, Willems B, Raymond G, Bourcier M, Cote J, Richer G.(1994).A long-term follow-up study of asymptomatic hepatitis B surface antigen-positive carriers in Montreal. *Gastroenterology*, 106(4):1000-1005.

[18] Lok AS, Lai CL, Wu PC, Leung EK.(1988).Long-term follow-up in a randomised controlled trial of recombinant alpha 2-interferon in Chinese patients with chronic hepatitis B infection. *Lancet*, 2(8606):298-302.

[19] Lok AS, Chung HT, Liu VW, Ma OC. (1993).Long-term follow-up of chronic hepatitis B patients treated with interferon alfa. *Gastroenterology*, 105(6):1833-1838.

[20] Carreno V, Castillo I, Molina J, Porres JC, Bartolome J.(1992).Long-term follow-up of hepatitis B chronic carriers who responded to interferon therapy. *J. Hepatol*, 15(1-2):102-106.

[21]   Fattovich G, Brollo L, Alberti A, Pontisso P, Giustina G, Realdi G.
        (1988).Long-term follow-up of anti-HBe-positive chronic active hepatitis
        B. *Hepatology*, 8(6):1651-1654.

[22]   Perrillo RP, Mason AL. (1994).Therapy for hepatitis B virus infection.
        Gastroenterol. Clin. North Am, 23(3):581-601.

[23]   Wong JB, Koff RS, Tine F, Pauker SG.(1995).Cost-effectiveness of
        interferon-alpha 2b treatment for hepatitis B e antigen-positive chronic
        hepatitis B. *Ann. Intern. Med*, 122(9):664-675.

[24]   Brugger SA, Oesterreicher C, Hofmann H, Kalhs P, Greinix HT, Muller
        C. (1997).Hepatitis B virus clearance by transplantation of bone marrow
        from hepatitis B immunised donor. *Lancet*, 349(9057):996-997.

[25]   Carr A, Cooper DA.(1997).Restoration of immunity to chronic hepatitis B
        infection in HIV-infected patient onprotease inhibitor. *Lancet*, 349(9057):
        995-996.

[26]   Malik AH, Lee WM.(2000).Chronic hepatitis B virus infection: treatment
        strategies for the next millennium. *Ann. Intern. Med*, 132(9):723-731.

[27]   Lok AS. (2002).Chronic hepatitis B. *N. Engl. J. Med*, 346(22):1682-1683.

[28]   Carreno V, Marcellin P, Hadziyannis S, Salmeron J, Diago M, Kitis GE,
        Vafiadis I, Schalm SW, Zahm F, Manzarbeitia F, Jimenez FJ, Quiroga
        JA.(1999).Retreatment of chronic hepatitis B e antigen-positive patients
        with recombinant interferon alfa-2a.The European Concerted Action on
        Viral Hepatitis (EUROHEP). *Hepatology*, 30(1):277-282.

[29]   Perrillo RP, Schiff ER, Davis GL, Bodenheimer HC, Jr., Lindsay K,
        Payne J, Dienstag JL, O'Brien C, Tamburro C, Jacobson IM, et al.
        (1990).A randomized, controlled trial of interferon alfa-2b alone and after
        prednisone withdrawal for the treatment of chronic hepatitis B.The
        Hepatitis Interventional Therapy Group. *N. Engl. J. Med*, 323(5):295-301.

[30]   Thomas HC, Lok AS, Carreno V, Farrell G, Tanno H, Perez V, Dusheiko
        GM, Cooksley G, Ryff JC.(1994).Comparative study of three doses of
        interferon-alpha 2a in chronic active hepatitis B.The International
        Hepatitis Trial Group. *J. Viral Hep*at, 1(2):139-148.

[31]   Korenman J, Baker B, Waggoner J, Everhart JE, Di Bisceglie AM,
        Hoofnagle JH.(1991).Long-term remission of chronic hepatitis B after
        alpha-interferon therapy. *Ann. Intern. Med*, 114(8):629-634.

[32]   Chen DK, Yim C, O'Rourke K, Krajden M, Wong DK, Heathcote
        EJ.(1999).Long-term follow-up of a randomized trial of interferon therapy
        for chronic hepatitis B in a predominantly homosexual male population. *J.
        Hepatol*, 30(4):557-563.

[33]   Ikeda K, Saitoh S, Suzuki Y, Kobayashi M, Tsubota A, Fukuda M, Koida
        I, Arase Y, Chayama K, Murashima N, Kumada H. (1998).Interferon
        decreases hepatocellular carcinogenesis in patients with cirrhosis caused
        by the hepatitis B virus: a pilot study. *Cancer*, 82(5):827-835.

[34]   Fattovich G, Giustina G, Realdi G, Corrocher R, Schalm SW. (1997).
        Long-term outcome of hepatitis B e antigen-positive patients with
        compensated cirrhosis treated with interferon alfa.European Concerted
        Action on Viral Hepatitis (EUROHEP). *Hepatology*, 26(5):1338-1342.

[35]   Brunetto MR, Oliveri F, Coco B, Leandro G, Colombatto P, Gorin JM,
        Bonino F. (2002).Outcome of anti-HBe positive chronic hepatitis B in
        alpha-interferon treated and untreated patients: a long term cohort study.
        J. Hepatol, 36(2):263-270.

[36]   Wong DK, Cheung AM, O'Rourke K, Naylor CD, Detsky AS, Heathcote
        J. (1993).Effect of alpha-interferon treatment in patients with hepatitis B e
        antigen-positive chronic hepatitis B.A meta-analysis. *Ann. Intern.* Med,
        119(4):312-323.

[37]   Lau DT, Everhart J, Kleiner DE, Park Y, Vergalla J, Schmid P, Hoofnagle
        JH. (1997).Long-term follow-up of patients with chronic hepatitis B
        treated with interferon alfa. *Gastroenterology*, 113(5):1660-1667.

[38]   Lin SM, Sheen IS, Chien RN, Chu CM, Liaw YF. (1999).Long-term
        beneficial effect of interferon therapy in patients with chronic hepatitis B
        virus infection. *Hepatology*, 29(3):971-975.

[39]   van Zonneveld M, Honkoop P, Hansen BE, Niesters HG, Murad SD, de
        Man RA, Schalm SW, Janssen HL. (2004).Long-term follow-up of alpha-
        interferon treatment of patients with chronic hepatitis B. *Hepatology*,
        39(3):804-810.

[40]   Niederau C, Heintges T, Lange S, Goldmann G, Niederau CM, Mohr L,
        Haussinger D. (1996).Long-term follow-up of HBeAg-positive patients
        treated with interferon alfa for chronic hepatitis B. *N. Engl. J. Med*, 334
        (22):1422-1427.

[41]   Yuen MF, Hui CK, Cheng CC, Wu CH, Lai YP, Lai CL. (2001).Long-
        term follow-up of interferon alfa treatment in Chinese patients with
        chronic hepatitis B infection: The effect on hepatitis B e antigen
        seroconversion and the development of cirrhosis-related complications.
        Hepatology, 34(1):139-145.

[42]   Lampertico P, Del Ninno E, Manzin A, Donato MF, Rumi MG, Lunghi G, Morabito A, Clementi M, Colombo M. (1997).A randomized, controlled trial of a 24-month course of interferon alfa 2b in patients with chronic hepatitis B who had hepatitis B virus DNA without hepatitis B e antigen in serum. *Hepatology*, 26(6):1621-1625.

[43]   Papatheodoridis GV, Manesis E, Hadziyannis SJ.(2001).The long-term outcome of interferon-alpha treated and untreated patients with HBeAg-negative chronic hepatitis B. *J. Hepatol*, 34(2):306-313.

[44]   Lau GK, Piratvisuth T, Luo KX, Marcellin P, Thongsawat S, Cooksley G, Gane E, Fried MW, Chow WC, Paik SW, Chang WY, Berg T, Flisiak R, McCloud P, Pluck N. (2005).Peginterferon Alfa-2a, lamivudine, and the combination for HBeAg-positive chronic hepatitis B. *N. Engl. J. Med*, 352(26):2682-2695.

[45]   Keeffe EB, Dieterich DT, Han SH, Jacobson IM, Martin P, Schiff ER, Tobias H, Wright TL. (2004).A treatment algorithm for the management of chronic hepatitis B virus infection in the United States. *Clin. Gastroenterol. Hepatol*, 2(2):87-106.

[46]   Manesis EK, Hadziyannis SJ. (2001).Interferon alpha treatment and retreatment of hepatitis B e antigen-negative chronic hepatitis B. *Gastroenterology*, 121(1):101-109.

[47]   Oliveri F, Santantonio T, Bellati G, Colombatto P, Mels GC, Carriero L, Dastoli G, Pastore G, Ideo G, Bonino F, Brunetto MR. (1999).Long term response to therapy of chronic anti-HBe-positive hepatitis B is poor independent of type and schedule of interferon. *Am. J. Gastroenterol*, 94 (5):1366-1372.

[48]   Johnson MA, Moore KH, Yuen GJ, Bye A, Pakes GE.(1999).Clinical pharmacokinetics of lamivudine. *Clin. Pharmacokinet*, 36(1):41-66.

[49]   Lai CL, Chien RN, Leung NWY, et al. (1998).A one-year trial of lamivudine for chronic hepatitis B. *N. Engl. J. Med*, 339:61-68.

[50]   Dienstag JL, Schiff ER, Wright TL, et al. (1999).Lamivudine as initial treatment for chronic hepatitis B in the United States. *N. Engl. J. Med*, 341:1256-1263.

[51]   Schalm SW, Heathcote J, Cianciara J, et al. (2000).Lamivudine and alpha interferon combination treatment of patients with chronic hepatitis B infection: a randomized trial. *Gut*, 46:562-568.

[52]   Schiff ER, Dienstag JL, Karayalcin S, et al. (2003).Lamivudine and 24 weeks of lamivudine/interferon combination therapy for hepatitis B e antigen-positive chronic hepatitis B in interferon nonresponders. *J. Hepatol*, 38:818-826.

[53]   Lok ASF, Lai C-L, Leung N, et al. (2003).Long-term safety of lamivudine treatment in patients with chronic hepatitis B. *Gastroenterology*, 125:1714-1722.

[54]   Lai CL, Dienstag J, Schiff E, et al. (2003).Prevalence and clinical correlates of YMDD variants during lamivudine therapy for patients with chronic hepatitis B. *Clin. Infect. Dis*, 36:687-696.

[55]   Chang TT, Lai CL, Chien RN, et al. (2004). Four years of lamivudine treatment in Chinese patients with chronic hepatitis C. *J. Gastroenterol. Hepatol*, 19:1276-1282.

[56]   Song BC, Suh DJ, Lee HC, et al. (2000).Hepatitis B e antigen seroconversion after lamivudine therapy is not durable in patients with chronic hepatitis B in Korea. *Hepatology*, 32:803-806.

[57]   Chien RN, Yeh CT, Tsai SL, et al. (2003).Determinants for sustained HBeAg response to lamivudine therapy. *Hepatology*, 38:1267-1273.

[58]   Liaw YF, Sung JJY, Chow WC, et al. (2004).Cirrhosis Asian Lamivudine Multicenter Study Group: Lamivudine for patients with chronic hepatitis B and advanced liver disease. *N. Engl. J. Med*, 351: 1521-1531.

[59]   Tassopoulos NC, Volpes R, Pastore G, et al. (1999).Efficacy of lamivudine in patients with hepatitis B e antigen-negative/hepatitis B virus DNA-positive (precore mutant) chronic hepatitis B. *Hepatology*, 29:889-896.

[60]   Hadziyannis SJ, Papatheodoridis GV, Dimou E, et al. (2000).Efficacy of long-term lamivudine monotherapy in patients with hepatitis B e antigen-negative chronic hepatitis B. *Hepatology*, 32:847-851.

[61]   Santantonio T, Mazzola M, Iacovazzi T et al. (2000).Long-term follow-up of patients with anti-HBe/HBV DNA-positive chronic hepatitis B treated for 12 months with lamivudine. *J. Hepatol*, 32(2): 300–306.

[62]   Dienstag JL, Schiff ER, Mitchell M et al. (1999).Extended lamivudine retreatment for chronic hepatitis B: maintenance of viral suppression after discontinuation of therapy. *Hepatology*, 30(4): 1082–1087.

[63]   Yang H, Westland CE, Delaney WE et al. (2002).Resistance surveillance in chronic hepatitis B patients treated with adefovir dipivoxil for up to 60 weeks. *Hepatology*, 36(2):464–473.

[64]   Perrillo R, Schiff E, Yoshida E et al. (2000).Adefovir dipivoxil for the treatment of lamivudine-resistant hepatitis B mutants. *Hepatology*, 32(1): 129–134.

[65]   Gilson RJ, Chopra KB, Newell AM et al. (1999).A placebo-controlled phase I/II study of adefovir dipivoxil in patients with chronic hepatitis B virus infection. *J. Viral Hep*at, 6(5): 387–395.

[66]   Marcellin P, Chang TT, Lim SG et al.(2003).Adefovir dipivoxil for the treatment of hepatitis B e antigen-positive chronic hepatitis B. *N. Engl. J. Med*, 348(9): 808–816.

[67]   Ono-Nita SK, Kato N, Shiratori Y et al. (1999).Susceptibility of lamivudine-resistant hepatitis B virus to other reverse transcriptase inhibitors. *J. Clin. Invest*, 103(12): 1635–1640.

[68]   Delaney WE, Edwards R, Colledge D et al. (2001).Cross-resistance testing of antihepadnaviral compounds using novel recombinant baculoviruses which encode drug-resistant strains of hepatitis B virus. *Antimicrob Agents Chemother*, 45(6):1705–1713.

[69]   Hadziyannis S, Tassopoulos N, Chang TT, et al. (2004).Three year study of adefovir dipivoxil (ADV) demonstrates sustained efficacy in presumed precore mutant chronic hepatitis B (CHB) patients in a long term safety and efficacy study (LTSES). *J. Hepatol*, 40(suppl 1):17.

[70]   Hadziyannis S, Tassopoulos N, Heathcote J, et al. (2003).Adefovir dipivoxil for the treatment of hepatitis B e antigen-negative chronic hepatitis B. *N. Engl. J. Med*, 348:800-807.

[71]   Hadziyannis S, Tassopoulos N, Heathcote J, et al. (2003).Long-term (96 weeks) adefovirdipivoxil in HbeAg negative chronic hepatitis results in significant virological,biochemical and histological improvement. *Hepatology*, 38(suppl 1):273A.

[72]   Perrillo RP, Hann HW, Mutimer D, et al. (2004).Adefovir dipivoxil added to ongoing lamivudine in chronic hepatitis B with YMDD mutant hepatitis B virus. *Gastroenterology*, 126:81-90.

[73]   Peters M, Hann, HW, Martin P, et al. (2004).Adefovir dipivoxil alone or in combination with lamivudine in patients with lamivudine-resistant chronic hepatitis B. *Gastroenterology*, 126:91-101.

[74]   de Man RA, Wolters LM, Nevens F et al. (2001).Safety and efficacy of oral entecavir given for 28 days in patients with chronic hepatitis B virus infection. *Hepatology*, 34(3): 578–582.

[75]   Tassopoulos N. (2001).Entecavir is effective in treating patients with chronic hepatitis B who have failed lamivudine therapy. *Hepatology* , 34(340A).

[76]   Glue P, Fang JW, Rouzier-Panis R et al. (2000). Pegylated interferonalpha2b: pharmacokinetics, pharmacodynamics, safety, and preliminary efficacy data. Hepatitis C Intervention Therapy Group. *Clin. Pharmacol. Ther*, 68(5): 556–567.

[77]   Zeuzem S, Feinman SV, Rasenack J et al. (2000).Peginterferon alfa-2a in patients with chronic hepatitis C. *N. Engl. J. Med*, 343(23): 1666–1672.

[78]   Heathcote EJ, Shiffman ML, Cooksley WG et al. (2000).Peginterferon alfa-2a in patients with chronic hepatitis C and cirrhosis. *N. Engl. J. Med*, 343 (23): 1673–1680.

[79]   Reddy KR, Wright TL, Pockros PJ et al. (2001).Efficacy and safety of pegylated (40-kd) interferon alpha-2a compared with interferon alpha-2a in noncirrhotic patients with chronic hepatitis C. *Hepatology*, 33(2): 433–438.

[80]   Lindsay KL, Trepo C, Heintges T et al. (2001).A randomized, doubleblind trial comparing pegylated interferon alfa-2b to interferon alfa-2b as initial treatment for chronic hepatitis C. *Hepatology*, 34(2): 395–403.

[81]   Cooksley WG, Piratvisuth T, Lee SD et al. (2003).Peginterferon alpha-2a (40 kDa): an advance in the treatment of hepatitis B e antigen-positive chronic hepatitis B. *J. Viral Hep*at, 10(4): 298–305.

[82]   Fried MW, Shiffman ML, Reddy KR, et al. (2002).Peginterferon alfa-2a plus ribavirin for chronic hepatitis C virus infection. *N. Engl. J. Med*, 347:975-982.

[83]   Alberti A, Brunetto MR, Colombo M, et al. (2002).Recent progress and new trends in the treatment of hepatitis B. *J. Med. Virol*, 67: 458-62.

[84]   Hanazaki K. (2004).Antiviral therapy for chronic hepatitis B: a review. *Curr. Drug Targets Inflamm. Allergy*, 3:63-70.

[85]   Wright TL.(2006).Introduction to chronic hepatitis B infection. *Am. J. Gastroenterol*, 101 (Suppl 1): S1-6.

[86]   King JK, Yeh SH, Lin MW, et al. (2002).Genetic polymorphisms in interferon pathway and response to interferon treatment in hepatitis B patients: A pilot study. *Hepatology*, 36: 1416-24.

[87]   Yu H, Zhu QR, Gu SQ et al. (2006).Relationship between IFN-gamma gene polymorphism and susceptibility to intrauterine HBV infection. *World J. Gastroenterol*, 12:2928-2931.

[88]   Kiepiela P, Leslie AJ, Honeyborne I, Ramduth D, Thobakgale C, Chetty S, Rathnavalu P, Moore C, Pfafferott KJ, Hilton L, Zimbwa P, Moore S, Allen T, Brander C, Addo MM, Altfeld M, James I, Mallal S, Bunce M, Barber LD, Szinger J, Day C, Klenerman P, Mullins J, Korber B, Coovadia HM, Walker BD, Goulder PJ.(2004).Dominant influence of HLA-B in mediating the potential co-evolution of HIV and HLA. *Nature*, 432(7018):769-775.

[89]   Stear MJ, Innocent GT, Buitkamp J. (2005).The evolution and maintenance of polymorphism in the major histocompatibility complex. *Vet. Immunol. Immunopathol*, 108(1-2):53-57.

[90]   Godkin A, Davenport M, Hill AV. (2005).Molecular analysis of HLA class II associations with hepatitis B virus clearance and vaccine nonresponsiveness. *Hepatology*, 41(6):1383-1390.

[91]   Kerkar N. (2005).Hepatitis B in children: complexities in management. *Pediatr. Transplant*, 9(5):685-691.

[92]   Villeneuve JP, Condreay LD, Willems B, Pomier-Layrargues G, Fenyves D, Bilodeau M, Leduc R, Peltekian K, Wong F, Margulies M, Heathcote EJ. (2000). Lamivudine treatment for decompensated cirrhosis resulting from chronic hepatitis B. *Hepatology*, 31(1):207-210.

[93]   Yao FY, Bass NM.(2000).Lamivudine treatment in patients with severely decompensated cirrhosis due to replicating hepatitis B infection. *J. Hepatol*, 33(2):301-307.

[94]   Kapoor D, Guptan RC, Wakil SM, Kazim SN, Kaul R, Agarwal SR, Raisuddin S, Hasnain SE, Sarin SK. (2000).Beneficial effects of lamivudine in hepatitis B virus-related decompensated cirrhosis. *J. Hepatol*, 33(2):308-312.

[95]   Perrillo RP, Wright T, Rakela J, Levy G, Schiff E, Gish R, Martin P, Dienstag J, Adams P, Dickson R, Anschuetz G, Bell S, Condreay L, Brown N. (2001).A multicenter United States-Canadian trial to assess lamivudine monotherapy before and after liver transplantation for chronic hepatitis B. *Hepatology*, 33(2):424-432.

[96]   Yao FY, Terrault NA, Freise C, Maslow L, Bass NM. (2001).Lamivudine treatment is beneficial in patients with severely decompensated cirrhosis and actively replicating hepatitis B infection awaiting liver transplantation: a comparative study using a matched, untreated cohort. *Hepatology*, 34(2):411-416.

[97]   Todo S, Demetris AJ, Van Thiel D, Teperman L, Fung JJ, Starzl TE.(1991).Orthotopic liver transplantation for patients with hepatitis B virus-related liver disease. *Hepatology*, 13(4):619-626.

[98]   O'Grady JG, Smith HM, Davies SE, Daniels HM, Donaldson PT, Tan KC, Portmann B, Alexander GJ, Williams R. (1992).Hepatitis B virus reinfection after orthotopic liver transplantation.serological and clinical implications. *J. Hepatol*, 14(1):104-111.

[99]   Davies SE, Portmann BC, O'Grady JG, Aldis PM, Chaggar K, Alexander GJ, Williams R. (1991).Hepatic histological findings after transplantation for chronic hepatitis B virus infection, including a unique pattern of fibrosing cholestatic hepatitis. *Hepatology*, 13(1):150-157.

[100]   Papatheodoridis GV, Sevastianos V, Burroughs AK.(2003).Prevention of and treatment for hepatitis B virus infection after liver transplantation in the nucleoside analogues era. *Am. J. Transplant*, 3(3):250-258.

[101]   Rosenau J, Bahr MJ, Tillmann HL, Trautwein C, Klempnauer J, Manns MP, Boker KHW. (2001). Lamivudine and low-dose hepatitis B immune globulin for prophylaxis of hepatitis B reinfection after liver transplantation possible role of mutations in the YMDD motif prior to transplantation as a risk factor for reinfection. *J. Hepatol*, 34(6):895-902.

[102]   Walsh KM, Woodall T, Lamy P, Wight DG, Bloor S, Alexander GJ.(2001).Successful treatment with adefovir dipivoxil in a patient with fibrosing cholestatic hepatitis and lamivudine resistant hepatitis B virus. *Gut*, 49(3):436-440.

[103]   Mutimer D, Feraz-Neto BH, Harrison R, O'Donnell K, Shaw J, Cane P, Pillay D. (2001).Acute liver graft failure due to emergence of lamivudine resistant hepatitis B virus: rapid resolution during treatment with adefovir. *Gut*, 49(6):860-863.

[104]   Wai CT, Prabhakaran K, Wee A, Lee YM, Dan YY, Sutedja DS, Mak K, Isaac J, Lee KH, Lee HL, Da Costa M, Lim SG. (2004).Adefovir dipivoxil as the rescue therapy for lamivudine-resistant hepatitis B post liver transplant. *Transplant. Proc*, 36(8):2313-2314.

[105]   Akay S, Karasu Z, Akyildiz M, Tokat Y. (2004).Adefovir treatment in posttransplant hepatitis B virus infection resistant to lamivudine plus hepatitis B virus immunoglobulin. *Transplant. Proc*, 36(9):2768-2770.

[106]   Seehofer D, Rayes N, Steinmuller T, Muller AR, Settmacher U, Neuhaus R, Radke C, Berg T, Hopf U, Neuhaus P. (2001).Occurrence and clinical outcome of lamivudine-resistant hepatitis B infection after liver transplantation. *Liver Transpl*, 7(11):976-982.

[107] Neff GW, O'Brien C B, Nery J, Shire N, Montalbano M, Ruiz P, Nery C, Safdar K, De Medina M, Tzakis AG, Schiff ER, Madariaga J. (2004). Outcomes in liver transplant recipients with hepatitis B virus: resistance and recurrence patterns from a large transplant center over the last decade. *Liver Transpl*, 10(11):1372-1378.

[108] Villeneuve JP, Durantel D, Durantel S, Westland C, Xiong S, Brosgart CL, Gibbs CS, Parvaz P, Werle B, Trepo C, Zoulim F. (2003).Selection of a hepatitis B virus strain resistant to adefovir in a liver transplantation patient. *J. Hepatol*, 39(6):1085-1089.

[109] Neff GW, Nery J, Lau DT, O'Brien CB, Duncan R, Shire NJ, Ruiz P, Nery C, Montalbano M, Muslu H, Safdar K, Schiff ER, Tzakis AG, Madariaga JR. (2004).Tenofovir therapy for lamivudine resistance following liver transplantation. *Ann. Pharmacother*, 38(12):1999-2004.

[110] Toniutto P, Fumo E, Caldato M, Apollonio L, Perin A, Pirisi M. (2004).Favourable outcome of adefovir-dipivoxil treatment in acute de novo hepatitis B after liver transplantation. *Transplantation*, 77(3):472-473.

[111] Samuel D, Muller R, Alexander G, Fassati L, Ducot B, Benhamou JP, Bismuth H. (1993).Liver transplantation in European patients with the hepatitis B surface antigen. *N. Engl. J. Med*, 329(25):1842-1847.

[112] Gonzalez RA, de la Mata M, de la Torre J, Mino G, Pera C, Pena J, Munoz E. (2000).Levels of HBV-DNA and HBsAg after acute liver allograft rejection treatment by corticoids and OKT3. *Clin. Transplant*, 14(3):208-211.

[113] Ho BM, So SK, Esquivel CO, Keeffe EB.(1997).Liver transplantation in Asian patients with chronic hepatitis B. *Hepatology*, 25(1):223-225.

[114] Teixeira R, Pastacaldi S, Papatheodoridis GV, Burroughs AK.(2000).Recurrent hepatitis C after liver transplantation. *J. Med. Virol*, 61(4):443-454.

[115] Mazzaferro V, Brunetto MR, Pasquali M, Regalia E, Pulvirenti A, Baratti D, Makowka L, Van Thiel D, Bonino F. (1997).Preoperative serum levels of wild-type and hepatitis B e antigen-negative hepatitis B virus (HBV) and graft infection after liver transplantation for HBV-related hepatocellular carcinoma. *J. Viral Hepat*, 4(4):235-242.

[116] Douglas DD, Rakela J, Wright TL, Krom RA, Wiesner RH.(1997).The clinical course of transplantation-associated de novo hepatitis B infection in the liver transplant recipient. *Liver Transpl. Surg*, 3(2):105-111.

[117] Terrault NA, Zhou S, Combs C, Hahn JA, Lake JR, Roberts JP, Ascher NL, Wright TL .(1996).Prophylaxis in liver transplant recipients using a fixed dosing schedule of hepatitis B immunoglobulin. *Hepatology*, 24(6):1327-1333.

[118] Muller R, Gubernatis G, Farle M, Niehoff G, Klein H, Wittekind C, Tusch G, Lautz HU, Boker K, Stangel W, et al. (1991).Liver transplantation in HBs antigen (HBsAg) carriers.prevention of hepatitis B virus (HBV) recurrence by passive immunization. *J. Hepatol*, 13(1):90-96.

[119] Samuel D, Bismuth A, Mathieu D, Arulnaden JL, Reynes M, Benhamou JP, Brechot C, Bismuth H.(1991).Passive immunoprophylaxis after liver transplantation in HBsAg-positive patients. *Lancet*, 337(8745):813-815.

[120] Rimoldi P, Belli LS, Rondinara GF, Alberti A, DeCarlis L, Minola E, Pirotta V, Meroni A, Romani F, Sansalone V, et al. (1993).Recurrent HBV/HDV infections under different immunoprophylaxis protocols. *Transplant. Proc*, 25(4):2675-2676.

[121] Steinmuller T, Seehofer D, Rayes N, Muller AR, Settmacher U, Jonas S, Neuhaus R, Berg T, Hopf U, Neuhaus P. (2002).Increasing applicability of liver transplantation for patients with hepatitis B-related liver disease. *Hepatology*, 35(6):1528-1535.

[122] Mohanty SR, Cotler SJ.(2005).Management of hepatitis B in liver transplant patients. *J. Clin. Gastroenterol*, 39(1):58-63.

[123] McGory RW, Ishitani MB, Oliveira WM, Stevenson WC, McCullough CS, Dickson RC, Caldwell SH, Pruett TL.(1996).Improved outcome of orthotopic liver transplantation for chronic hepatitis B cirrhosis with aggressive passive immunization. *Transplantation*, 61(9):1358-1364.

[124] Konig V, Hopf U, Neuhaus P, Bauditz J, Schmidt CA, Blumhardt G, Bechstein WO, Neuhaus R, Lobeck H. (1994).Long-term follow-up of hepatitis B virus-infected recipients after orthotopic liver transplantation. *Transplantation*, 58(5):553-559.

[125] Samuel D, Bismuth A, Serres C, Arulnaden JL, Reynes M, Benhamou JP, Brechot C, Bismuth H. (1991).HBV infection after liver transplantation in HBsAg positive patients: experience with long-term immunoprophylaxis. *Transplant. Proc*, 23(1 Pt 2):1492-1494.

[126] Sawyer RG, McGory RW, Gaffey MJ, McCullough CC, Shephard BL, Houlgrave CW, Ryan TS, Kuhns M, McNamara A, Caldwell SH, Abdulkareem A, Pruett TL.(1998).Improved clinical outcomes with liver transplantation for hepatitis B-induced chronic liver failure using passive immunization. *Ann. Surg*, 227(6):841-850.

[127] Cooreman MP, Leroux-Roels G, Paulij WP. (2001).Vaccine- and hepatitis B immune globulin-induced escape mutations of hepatitis B virus surface antigen. *J. Biomed. Sci,* 8(3):237-247.

[128] McMahon G, Ehrlich PH, Moustafa ZA, McCarthy LA, Dottavio D, Tolpin MD, Nadler PI, Ostberg L.(1992).Genetic alterations in the gene encoding the major HBsAg: DNA and immunological analysis of recurrent HBsAg derived from monoclonal antibody-treated liver transplant patients. *Hepatology,* 15(5):757-766.

[129] Galun E, Terrault NA, Eren R, Zauberman A, Nussbaum O, Terkieltaub D, Zohar M, Buchnik R, Ackerman Z, Safadi R, Ashur Y, Misrachi S, Liberman Y, Rivkin L, Dagan S. (2007).Clinical evaluation (Phase I) of a human monoclonal antibody against hepatitis C virus: Safety and antiviral activity. *J. Hepatol,* 46(1):37-44.

[130] Buti M, Mas A, Prieto M, Casafont F, Gonzalez A, Miras M, Herrero JI, Jardi R, Cruz de Castro E, Garcia-Rey C. (2003).A randomized study comparing lamivudine monotherapy after a short course of hepatitis B immune globulin (HBIg) and lamivudine with long-term lamivudine plus HBIg in the prevention of hepatitis B virus recurrence after liver transplantation. *J. Hepatol,* 38(6):811-817.

[131] Dumortier J, Chevallier P, Scoazec JY, Berger F, Boillot O. (2003).Combined lamivudine and hepatitis B immunoglobulin for the prevention of hepatitis B recurrence after liver transplantation: long-term results. *Am. J. Transplant,* 3(8):999-1002.

[132] Dienstag JL, Perrillo RP, Schiff ER, Bartholomew M, Vicary C, Rubin M. (1995).A preliminary trial of lamivudine for chronic hepatitis B infection. *N. Engl. J. Med,* 333(25):1657-1661.

[133] Marzano A, Salizzoni M, Debernardi-Venon W, Smedile A, Franchello A, Ciancio A, Gentilcore E, Piantino P, Barbui AM, David E, Negro F, Rizzetto M. (2001).Prevention of hepatitis B virus recurrence after liver transplantation in cirrhotic patients treated with lamivudine and passive immunoprophylaxis. *J. Hepatol,* 34(6):903-910.

[134] Grellier L, Mutimer D, Ahmed M, Brown D, Burroughs AK, Rolles K, McMaster P, Beranek P, Kennedy F, Kibbler H, McPhillips P, Elias E, Dusheiko G. (1996).Lamivudine prophylaxis against reinfection in liver transplantation for hepatitis B cirrhosis. *Lancet,* 348(9036):1212-1215.

[135]   Markowitz JS, Martin P, Conrad AJ, Markmann JF, Seu P, Yersiz H, Goss
        JA, Schmidt P, Pakrasi A, Artinian L, Murray NG, Imagawa DK, Holt C,
        Goldstein LI, Stribling R, Busuttil RW.(1998).Prophylaxis against
        hepatitis B recurrence following liver transplantation using combination
        lamivudine and hepatitis B immune globulin. *Hepatology*, 28(2):585-589.
[136]   Lo CM, Cheung ST, Lai CL, Liu CL, Ng IO, Yuen MF, Fan ST, Wong J.
        (2001).Liver transplantation in Asian patients with chronic hepatitis B
        using lamivudine prophylaxis. *Ann. Surg*, 233(2):276-281.
[137]   Seehofer D, Rayes N, Naumann U, Neuhaus R, Muller AR, Tullius SG,
        Berg T, Steinmuller T, Bechstein WO, Neuhaus P. (2001).Preoperative
        antiviral treatment and postoperative prophylaxis in HBV-DNA positive
        patients undergoing liver transplantation. *Transplantation*, 72(8):1381-
        1385.
[138]   Fontana RJ, Keeffe EB, Carey W, Fried M, Reddy R, Kowdley KV,
        Soldevila-Pico C, McClure LA, Lok AS.(2002).Effect of lamivudine
        treatment on survival of 309 North American patients awaiting liver
        transplantation for chronic hepatitis B. *Liver Transpl*, 8(5):433-439.
[139]   Andreone P, Biselli M, Gramenzi A, Cursaro C, Morelli MC, Sama C,
        Lorenzini S, Spinucci G, Porzio F, Felline F, Di Giammarino L, Bernardi
        M. (2002).Efficacy of lamivudine therapy for advanced liver disease in
        patients with precore mutant hepatitis B virus infection awaiting liver
        transplantation. *Transplantation*, 74(8):1119-1124.
[140]   Fontana RJ, Hann HW, Perrillo RP, Vierling JM, Wright T, Rakela J,
        Anschuetz G, Davis R, Gardner SD, Brown NA. (2002). Determinants of
        early mortality in patients with decompensated chronic hepatitis B treated
        with antiviral therapy. *Gastroenterology*, 123(3):719-727.
[141]   Liaw YF, Leung NW, Chang TT, Guan R, Tai DI, Ng KY, Chien RN,
        Dent J, Roman L, Edmundson S, Lai CL. (2000).Effects of extended
        lamivudine therapy in Asian patients with chronic hepatitis B. Asia
        Hepatitis Lamivudine Study Group. *Gastroenterology*, 119(1):172-180.
[142]   Leung NW, Lai CL, Chang TT, Guan R, Lee CM, Ng KY, Lim SG, Wu
        PC, Dent JC, Edmundson S, Condreay LD, Chien RN. (2001).Extended
        lamivudine treatment in patients with chronic hepatitis B enhances
        hepatitis B e antigen seroconversion rates: results after 3 years of therapy.
        Hepatology, 33(6): 1527-1532.

[143] Stuyver LJ, Locarnini SA, Lok A, Richman DD, Carman WF, Dienstag JL, Schinazi RF. (2001).Nomenclature for antiviral-resistant human hepatitis B virus mutations in the polymerase region. *Hepatology*, 33(3):751-757.

[144] Liaw YF.(2003).Results of lamivudine trials in Asia. *J Hepatol*, 39 Suppl 1:S111-S115

[145] Zoulim F. (2002).A preliminary benefit-risk assessment of lamivudine for the treatment of chronic hepatitis B virus infection. *Drug Saf*, 25(7):497-510.

[146] Mutimer D, Dusheiko G, Barrett C, Grellier L, Ahmed M, Anschuetz G, Burroughs A, Hubscher S, Dhillon AP, Rolles K, Elias E. (2000).Lamivudine without HBIg for prevention of graft reinfection by hepatitis B: long-term follow-up. *Transplantation*, 70(5):809-815.

[147] Vierling JM.(2005).Management of HBV Infection in Liver Transplantation Patients. *Int. J. Med. Sci*, 2(1):41-49.

[148] Malkan G, Cattral MS, Humar A, Al Asghar H, Greig PD, Hemming AW, Levy GA, Lilly LB. (2000).Lamivudine for hepatitis B in liver transplantation: a single-center experience. *Transplantation*, 69(7):1403-1407.

[149] Naoumov NV, Lopes AR, Burra P, Caccamo L, Iemmolo RM, de Man RA, Bassendine M, O'Grady JG, Portmann BC, Anschuetz G, Barrett CA, Williams R, Atkins M.(2001).Randomized trial of lamivudine versus hepatitis B immunoglobulin for long-term prophylaxis of hepatitis B recurrence after liver transplantation. *J. Hepatol*, 34(6):888-894.

[150] Mutimer D, Pillay D, Dragon E, Tang H, Ahmed M, O'Donnell K, Shaw J, Burroughs N, Rand D, Cane P, Martin B, Buchan S, Boxall E, Barmat S, Gutekunst K, McMaster P, Elias E. (1999).High pre-treatment serum hepatitis B virus titre predicts failure of lamivudine prophylaxis and graft re-infection after liver transplantation. *J. Hepatol*, 30(4):715-721.

[151] Angus PW, McCaughan GW, Gane EJ, Crawford DH, Harley H. (2000).Combination low-dose hepatitis B immune globulin and lamivudine therapy provides effective prophylaxis against posttransplantation hepatitis B. *Liver Transpl*, 6(4):429-433.

[152] Yao FY, Osorio RW, Roberts JP, Poordad FF, Briceno MN, Garcia-Kennedy R, Gish RR. (1999).Intramuscular hepatitis B immune globulin combined with lamivudine for prophylaxis against hepatitis B recurrence after liver transplantation. *Liver Transpl. Surg*, 5(6):491-496.

[153] Yoshida EM, Erb SR, Partovi N, Scudamore CH, Chung SW, Frighetto L, Eggen HJ, Steinbrecher UP.(1999).Liver transplantation for chronic hepatitis B infection with the use of combination lamivudine and low-dose hepatitis B immune globulin. *Liver Transpl. Surg*, 5(6):520-525.

[154] McCaughan GW, Spencer J, Koorey D, Bowden S, Bartholomeusz A, Littlejohn M, Verran D, Chui AK, Sheil AG, Jones RM, Locarnini SA, Angus PW. (1999).Lamivudine therapy in patients undergoing liver transplantation for hepatitis B virus precore mutant-associated infection: high resistance rates in treatment of recurrence but universal prevention if used as prophylaxis with very low dose hepatitis B immune globulin. *Liver Transpl. Surg*, 5(6):512-519.

[155] Han SH, Ofman J, Holt C, King K, Kunder G, Chen P, Dawson S, Goldstein L, Yersiz H, Farmer DG, Ghobrial RM, Busuttil RW, Martin P. (2000).An efficacy and cost-effectiveness analysis of combination hepatitis B immune globulin and lamivudine to prevent recurrent hepatitis B after orthotopic liver transplantation compared with hepatitis B immune globulin monotherapy. *Liver Transpl*, 6(6):741-748.

[156] Hadziyannis SJ, Tassopoulos NC, Heathcote EJ, Chang TT, Kitis G, Rizzetto M, Marcellin P, Lim SG, Goodman Z, Wulfsohn MS, Xiong S, Fry J, Brosgart CL. (2003).Adefovir dipivoxil for the treatment of hepatitis B e antigen-negative chronic hepatitis B. *N. Engl. J. Med*, 348(9):800-807.

[157] Benhamou Y, Bochet M, Thibault V, Calvez V, Fievet MH, Vig P, Gibbs CS, Brosgart C, Fry J, Namini H, Katlama C, Poynard T. (2001).Safety and efficacy of adefovir dipivoxil in patients co-infected with HIV-1 and lamivudine-resistant hepatitis B virus: an open-label pilot study. *Lancet*, 358(9283):718-723.

[158] Deeks SG, Collier A, Lalezari J, Pavia A, Rodrigue D, Drew WL, Toole J, Jaffe HS, Mulato AS, Lamy PD, Li W, Cherrington JM, Hellmann N, Kahn J. (1997).The safety and efficacy of adefovir dipivoxil, a novel anti-human immunodeficiency virus (HIV) therapy, in HIV-infected adults: a randomized, double-blind, placebo-controlled trial. *J. Infect. Dis*, 176(6):1517-1523.

[159]   Schiff ER, Lai CL, Hadziyannis S, Neuhaus P, Terrault N, Colombo M, Tillmann HL, Samuel D, Zeuzem S, Lilly L, Rendina M, Villeneuve JP, Lama N, James C, Wulfsohn MS, Namini H, Westland C, Xiong S, Choy GS, Van Doren S, Fry J, Brosgart CL.(2003).Adefovir dipivoxil therapy for lamivudine-resistant hepatitis B in pre- and post-liver transplantation patients. *Hepatology*, 38(6):1419-1427.

[160]   Lo CM, Liu CL, Lau GK, Chan SC, Ng IO, Fan ST. (2005).Liver transplantation for chronic hepatitis B with lamivudine-resistant YMDD mutant using add-on adefovir dipivoxil plus lamivudine. *Liver Transpl*, 11(7):807-813.

[161]   Westland CE, Yang H, Delaney WE 4th, Wulfsohn M, Lama N, Gibbs CS, Miller MD, Fry J, Brosgart CL, Schiff ER, Xiong S.(2005).Activity of adefovir dipivoxil against all patterns of lamivudine-resistant hepatitis B viruses in patients. *J. Viral Hepat,*12(1):67-73.

[162]   Fung SK, Andreone P, Han SH, Rajender Reddy K, Regev A, Keeffe EB, Hussain M, Cursaro C, Richtmyer P, Marrero JA, Lok AS. (2005).Adefovir-resistant hepatitis B can be associated with viral rebound and hepatic decompensation. *J. Hepatol*, 43(6):937-943.

[163]   Fung SK, Chae HB, Fontana RJ, Conjeevaram H, Marrero J, Oberhelman K, Hussain M, Lok AS.(2006).Virologic response and resistance to adefovir in patients with chronic hepatitis B. *J. Hepatol*, 44(2):283-290.

[164]   Perrillo R, Rakela J, Dienstag J, Levy G, Martin P, Wright T, Caldwell S, Schiff E, Gish R, Villeneuve JP, Farr G, Anschuetz G, Crowther L, Brown N. (1999).Multicenter study of lamivudine therapy for hepatitis B after liver transplantation.lamivudine Transplant Group. *Hepatology*, 29(5):1581-1586.

[165]   Rayes N, Seehofer D, Hopf U, Neuhaus R, Naumann U, Bechstein WO, Neuhaus P. (2001).Comparison of famciclovir and lamivudine in the long-term treatment of hepatitis B infection after liver transplantation. *Transplantation*, 71(1):96-101.

[166]   Fontana RJ, Hann HW, Wright T, Everson G, Baker A, Schiff ER, Riely C, Anschuetz G, Riker-Hopkins M, Brown N. (2001).A multicenter study of lamivudine treatment in 33 patients with hepatitis B after liver transplantation. *Liver Transpl*, 7(6):504-510.

[167]   Honkoop P, De Man RA. (2003).Entecavir: a potent new antiviral drug for hepatitis B. Expert Opin. Investig Drugs, 12(4):683-688.

[168]   Wolters LM, Hansen BE, Niesters HG, DeHertogh D, de Man RA. (2002).Viral dynamics during and after entecavir therapy in patients with chronic hepatitis B. *J. Hepatol*, 37(1):137-144.

[169]   Kuo A, Dienstag JL, Chung RT. (2004).Tenofovir disoproxil fumarate for the treatment of lamivudine-resistant hepatitis B. *Clin. Gastroenterol. Hepatol*, 2(3):266-272.

[170]   Van Bommel F, Schernick A, Hopf U, Berg T. (2003).Tenofovir disoproxil fumarate exhibits strong antiviral effect in a patient with lamivudine-resistant severe hepatitis B reactivation. *Gastroenterology*, 124(2):586-587.

[171]   Van Bommel F, Wunsche T, Schurmann D, Berg T. (2002).Tenofovir treatment in patients with lamivudine-resistant hepatitis B mutants strongly affects viral replication. *Hepatology*, 36(2):507-508.

[172]   Taltavull TC, Chahri N, Verdura B, Gornals J, Lopez C, Casanova A, Canas C, Figueras J, Casais LA.(2005).Successful treatment with tenofovir in a child C cirrhotic patient with lamivudine-resistant hepatitis B virus awaiting liver transplantation. Post-transplant results. *Transpl. Int*, 18(7):879-883.

Conclusion

The Hepatitis B virus is a DNA virus that can cause both acute and chronic liver disease in humans. If cirrhosis and liver failure develops, the definitive treatment of choice remains orthotopic liver transplantation (OLT). In the past, recurrence of HBV was common following OLT leading to unacceptable rates of graft loss and increased morbidity and mortality.

With the advent of new antiviral therapy, it should be possible to prevent recurrence in most, if not all, post-transplant patients. Ideally, the antiviral regimen should be robust and prevent breakthrough mutations. In decompensated cirrhotic patients, the use of combination therapy has the advantage of reducing the risk of escape mutations. A prudent approach in preventing recurrence may be the implication of combination antiviral therapy in the post-transplant setting as well. This remains an unanswered question. As discussed above, most studies using combination therapy have been small; although favorable results are seen.

Fortunately, for those who have already developed recurrent disease, newer agents, either alone or in combination, are able to achieve significant reductions in the HBV DNA level and normalization of transaminases.

A pending controversy is the duration of HBIG therapy. While the use of HBIG infusions is universally accepted as advantageous in the perioperative setting, the use of combination oral agents may make it possible to stop this costly therapy after a short period of time or avoid it entirely. This remains a contentious issue that requires further studies before a definitive recommendation can be made.

Future Prospects

HBV infection is closely related to the development of liver diseases. However, the pathogenesis of HBV-related HCC is incompletely clarified. HBx plays a crucial role in HCC occurrence, invasion and metastasis. We suggest that antibody to hepatitis B x antigen (anti-HBx) should be monitored in predicting early diagnosis of LC and HCC. Some molecular approaches, such as antisense, oligonucleotides, ribozymes, RNA interference targeting HBV mRNA, are available in antiviral therapies. The intracellular antibody technique and immune therapy by dendritic cells are potentially used in the future antiviral therapies.

At present, the exact pathogenesis of HBV infection is still not completely clarified. In the research, some key issues remain to undergoing, such as the HBV variants and genome instability, and immunopathogenesis, etc. In our opinion, to evolve the field over the next 5-10 years, we should pay more attention to the research of HBV molecular virology. As HBV genotypes have been alleged to be associated with the development of LC and HCC, determining the genotype could be helpful to predict the outcome of antiviral therapy. HBV carriers are at high risk for the development of HCC, however, there are no reliable biomarkers that can identify such high-risk carriers. Maybe we should make more efforts to identify new biomarkers for early diagnosis and assessment of disease progression. As the presence of anti-HBx is known to correlate to the well-established serological marker, monitoring anti-HBx may be available for diagnosis and prognosis of LC and HCC. In viral-related cirrhosis, HBV and HCV or HIV coinfections increase the HCC risk. Thus, the research of the coinfection should be strengthened. All the outcomes provide us the knowledge for molecular approaches, such as antisense, oligonucleotides, ribozymes, RNA interference targeting HBV mRNA, which may be potentially used in antiviral therapy. Additionally, intracellular antibody technique or dendritic cell based therapy are possibly applied in the future therapy. Investigation of treatment vaccine for HBV infection is undergoing on, which is hopeful to apply in clinic in near future. Moreover, the prevention for HBV infection is very important. Not only the vaccination is carried out but also the effect of immunoreaction on the body should be monitored after the vaccination.

Index

N

O

R

S

T

U

V